MAKING SENSE OF MEDICAL ETHICS

MAKING SENSE OF MEDICAL ETHICS

A HANDS-ON GUIDE

Alan G. Johnson
MA MB MChir DSc(Hon) FRCS(Eng)
Emeritus Professor of Surgery at the University of Sheffield,
Sheffield, UK

Paul R.V. Johnson
MBChB MA MD FRCS(Eng) FRCS(Edin) FRCS(Paed Surg)
Reader in Paediatric Surgery at the University of Oxford,
Honorary Consultant Paediatric Surgeon at the John Radcliffe
Hospital, Oxford, UK, and Director of the Oxford Pancreatic
Islet Transplant Programme

Hodder Arnold

A MEMBER OF THE HODDER HEADLINE GROUP

First published in Great Britain in 2006 by
Hodder Arnold, an imprint of Hodder Education and a member of the Hodder
Headline Group, 338 Euston Road, London NW1 3BH

http://www.hoddereducation.com

Distributed in the United States of America by
Oxford University Press Inc.,
198 Madison Avenue, New York, NY 10016
Oxford is a registered trademark of Oxford University Press

British Library Cataloguing in Publication Data
A catalogue record for this book is available from the British Library

Library of Congress Cataloging-in-Publication Data
A catalog record for this book is available from the Library of Congress

ISBN-10   0 340 925 590
ISBN-13   978 0 340 925 591

1 2 3 4 5 6 7 8 9 10

Commissioning Editor:	Sara Purdy
Project Editor:	Jane Tod
Production Controller:	Lindsay Smith
Cover Design:	Nichola Smith
Cartoon Illustrations	Patrick Elliott
Indexer:	Lawrence Errington

Typeset in 10.5/13 Rotis Serif by Charon Tec Ltd (A Macmillan Company),
Chennai, India
www.charontec.com
Printed and bound in Italy

What do you think about this book? Or any other Hodder Arnold title?
Please visit our website: www.hoddereducation.com

*To Esther and Hilary whose support and
encouragement have been invaluable.*

ABOUT THE AUTHORS

Alan Johnson read Natural Sciences including History and Philosophy of Science at Cambridge University before completing clinical studies at University College Hospital, London. His interest in medical ethics started as an undergraduate. After surgical training in and around London, he was appointed Senior Lecturer in surgery at Charing Hospital Medical School in 1971. Here, with Brian Bliss, he pioneered the teaching of ethics by regular student seminars during clinical attachments, at a time when there was very little ethics teaching in British medical schools. This led to his first book on the subject. (Bliss and Johnson, 1975, *Aims and motives in Clinical Medicine.* Sevenoaks: Pittman Medical) He was also chairman of the Research Ethics Committee. In 1979, he was appointed Professor of Surgery at Sheffield University, in 1990 he published *Pathways in Medical Ethics* (London: Arnold) and in 1998 chaired the working party for the Senate of Surgery on *The Surgeons Duty Of Care.* He has also chaired Steering and Data Monitoring and Ethics Committees for Medical Research Council clinical trials. In 1993–4 he was President of the Association of Surgeons of Great Britain and Ireland and from 1998–2002, Chairman of the Standing Medical Advisory Committee to the Secretary of State for Health, which faced many issues of the priorities and fair distribution of health care. He has lectured on medical ethics to students and postgraduates, as well as lay audiences, in many countries and continues to advise and teach in the University of Sheffield.

Paul Johnson graduated in medicine from the University of Leicester Medical School and did his Basic Surgical training in Leicester and Derby. He then spent 3 years in the field of pancreatic islet transplantation for which he was awarded a Doctorate and a Hunterian Professorship of the Royal College of Surgeons of England. He underwent Higher Surgical

Training in Paediatric Surgery in Oxford, in Great Ormand Street Hospital, London and The Royal Children's Hospital, Melbourne, Australia. In 2001, he was appointed Reader in Paediatric Surgery at the University of Oxford, Honorary Paediatric Surgeon at the John Radcliffe Hospital, Oxford and a Fellow of St. Edmund's Hall. He is actively involved in teaching undergraduates embryology, and varied aspects of paediatric surgery and is Clinical Tutor at St. Edmund Hall. His clinical practice regularly involves dealing with the ethical dilemmas of neonatal surgery and antenatal counselling, and his research programme in pancreatic islet-cell transplantation brings him face to face with the ethics of transplantation and the new challenges of stem-cell biology.

CONTENTS

PREFACE

Dame Janet Smith, chair of the Shipman Inquiry, called for a greater emphasis on ensuring that medical students are aware of professional ethics early in their training, and even suggested that medical students who fail to demonstrate 'ethical sense' should not be allowed to qualify (Smith, 2005). On the other hand, David Sokol points out that it is 'unrealistic to expect medical students to learn more than the bare bones of the subject', given that their curriculum is already overloaded, or to expect junior doctors to undergo extensive training in medical ethics, while working full-time (Sokol, 2005). This book is written to resolve this paradox. Asking students to learn rules, without understanding how or why they came about, goes completely against current methods of medical education. Instead, to make sense of this difficult subject, we need to highlight the key issues, clarify confusions, and provide a clear and logical framework for ethical decision making.

We start by defining the subject and exploring some of the misunderstandings surrounding medical ethics. We then outline the main ethical theories and explain how the different value systems and world-views inform ethical thinking and decision-making. Our approach throughout, however, is practical rather than purely theoretical, and the examples throughout the book are nearly all based on real clinical situations. We then discuss if, and how, a professional consensus can be reached and identify how law and ethics interact. As well as analysing in detail the five main ethical principles, we show that they are often in 'competition'. We suggest ways in which this competition can be resolved and how ethical priorities can be established. We demonstrate the use of an algorithm in making ethical decisions in a variety of different situations.

The last two chapters emphasize particular ethical dilemmas faced by students (including examinations!), and ask 'What makes an ethical doctor?' Throughout the book, we challenge readers to examine their own values and to be clear why we even care for sick people in the first place.

The book does not aim to cover every topic systematically; some are mentioned in several different sections to illustrate different principles and algorithms, so the index and further reading guides need to be used. Although the book is aimed primarily at medical students and junior doctors, we have made it accessible to many other health care and lay groups. We hope we have not only made sense of medical ethics, but also stimulated a long-term practical interest in this engrossing and important subject.

Alan G Johnson, Sheffield
Paul RV Johnson, Oxford

ACKNOWLEDGEMENTS

We are very grateful to the following for their help and advice: Ruth Bird (medical student), Mrs Vidya P Chandran, Esther Johnson, Dr Robert Peck, Dr Ziaur Rahman, Dr Mandy Sharpe and Della Oldham. We are especially indebted to Patrick Elliott for enlivening the text with his inimitable illustrations.

'Sapere Aude – Dare to be wise.'

(Horace)

'The fear of the Lord is the beginning of wisdom.'
(Old Jewish Proverb)

'The patients that enter our department have feelings, opinions, needs and rights and we are here to meet them in the best possible way. In the operating department our patients are generally feeling extremely vulnerable, so we act as their advocate, assuming responsibility for their wellbeing and dignity.'

(Philosophy, Operating Theatres,
The John Radcliffe Hospital, Oxford)

WHAT IS IT ALL ABOUT?

The morning medical ward round has just started and the patient in the first bed of a six-bedded ward asks the team whether his HIV test was positive. Having just received the positive result before the round, do we lie to preserve the patient's confidentiality or answer truthfully and risk his fellow patients shunning him and spreading the news around

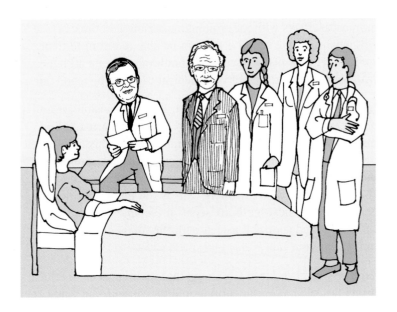

the neighbourhood? In the next ward a frightened woman, whose first language is not English, refuses to give consent for an urgent, possibly life-saving operation until she has discussed it with her husband who is abroad and cannot be contacted. Do we go ahead against her will to save her life? What right has her husband to make the decision? Did she really understand the importance and urgency of the situation when you explained it to her?

At lunchtime, accompanied by a quickly snatched sandwich, you attend a seminar where a research fellow is talking about the use of pancreatic stem cells for treating children with insulin-dependent diabetes. The cells are taken from aborted foetuses. Are people then 'killing' one life in order to save another? After lunch your mind begins to ponder the relative values of foetuses and children and what rights we all have. In the afternoon you attend a busy outpatient clinic where the last patient has cancer which has spread despite standard chemotherapy. The consultant is considering whether to use a recently licensed highly expensive drug, which has not yet been shown to be effective in this situation. It could give the patient more side-effects without prolonging her life and the expense will mean that the hospital will not be able to afford to treat some other patients with curable conditions. We are all left wondering how the delivery of medical care can be made fair.

In the evening you chill-out in front of the television set and a documentary reports that Dr Harold Shipman started killing his patients while he was a very junior doctor. This is followed by a programme about the German concentration camps during the Second World War and the medical experiments conducted on Jewish prisoners. This is too much for one day and even a medical textbook seems preferable! So you switch off the TV and soon fall asleep with the textbook open and unread on your lap.

All day you have faced situations that involve medical ethical principles such as truth, confidentiality, consent, the value of human life from conception to human adulthood, fairness, autonomy of research subjects and doctors' motivation. Before considering these practical dilemmas, we must ask some more fundamental questions about peoples' values, how we derive ethical principles, and how we resolve the apparent conflicts between them.

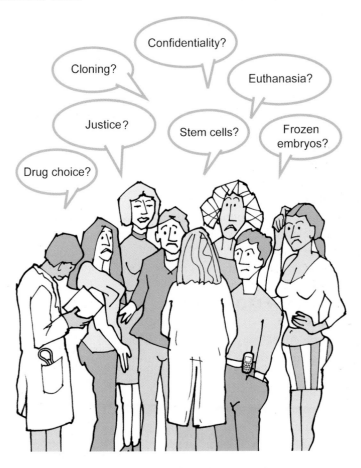

Ethical guidance is not intended as an oppressive legal burden trying to catch us out at every turn, although of course there must be limits to doctors' behaviour, the breach of which leads to sanctions.

IS IT ETHICAL?

This question is asked hundreds of times a year in surgeries, wards, research laboratories, health planning departments, government committees and in the media. Of course it cannot be answered without knowing the exact details of the particular situation and thinking clearly through all the issues. Moreover, the question is meaningless without defining the ethical framework against which the action is being assessed. If your ethical obligation is to 'perfect' the human race, and you believe that the end justifies the means, then the destruction of disabled children is entirely consistent with your ethics. If, on the other hand, the sanctity of human life is one of your key ethical principles, you will be appalled by that and have real conflicts when it comes to deciding priorities of care and how far to go to maintain the life of someone who has severe disability.

In practice, the question 'Is it ethical?' usually means: 'Does it fit with the accepted norms of current medical practice or the guidelines governing clinical research?'

ETHICS OR MORALS?

The word 'ethics' may conjure up a theoretical concept detached from reality, with 'thinkers in ivory towers' debating philosophical concepts. To the academic ethicist, the word 'ethics' means the philosophical study of the moral values of human contact and the rules and principles that ought to govern it. An alternative name for this is moral philosophy. In fact 'ethics' is derived from Greek and 'morals' is a Latin word for the same idea. The word 'morals' is more down to earth and 'moral or immoral' seems more practical then 'ethical or unethical'. 'Ethics' refers to a framework or set of principles, whereas 'morals' tends to be used more about individual behaviour and often has an emotional dimension.

> The purpose of medical ethics is to clarify the moral issues, give principles on which to act and guidance in the details of making the right decisions.

DEFINITIONS

The following are two examples of the many definitions of medical ethics:

> *Obligations of a moral nature that govern the practice of medicine.*
>
> **(Dunstan, 1974)**

> *The study of moral ideals, rules and codes of conduct that govern the behaviour of medical professionals.*
>
> **(Grenz and Smith, 2003, page 74)**

Both definitions carry the three concepts of duty, morals and governance.

Duty

The practice of ethics is not a hobby, like golf or playing the violin, which doctors can choose and then discontinue when they are too busy. Someone joining the medical profession takes on certain obligations and patterns of behaviour, the breaking of which can even lead to deregistration.

Morals

Moral issues involve life and death, healing and harm, justice and integrity. There has been a tendency in the past to confuse the terms ethics and etiquette. Etiquette is concerned with traditions and politeness of behaviour between colleagues that make for the smooth running of the profession – more social than of great significance – and has, at times, been used in the past to cover up poor practice.

Governance

Moral duties should govern the practice of medicine, not just be tagged on behind. Sometimes new scientific advances or treatments have been introduced and only afterwards have the rightness and control of their use been discussed. By the time an ethical decision has been made the procedure is already well established. One of the positive things about the Human Genome Project was that from the beginning, a budget was identified to study the possible implications of the findings. Similarly in many countries, regulations have been introduced to control the extension of experimental cloning techniques to human reproductive cloning.

The practice of medicine cannot be divorced from its ethics at any stage. Even disciplines that do not involve direct patient contact, such as pathology, have ethical constraints, as the Alder Hey Inquiry (Royal Liverpool Children's Inquiry, 2001) has reminded us.

ETHICS IN OTHER AREAS OF LIFE

In one sense there is no such thing as 'medical ethics', if what is meant by that is ethics exclusive to medicine. It is easy to think that medicine is unique from all other areas of activity in requiring ethical control because it is concerned with people's lives and health. But decisions in many other jobs also have effects in these areas. Business ethics, for example, can allow cigarette companies to make huge amounts of money while being responsible for the deaths of 350 people a day in the UK. On the other hand, business ethics can ensure fair trade so that the producers in developing countries get a fair share of the rewards. The 'ethics of war' put the conflicts of medical ethics in the shade: many lives may be sacrificed for a political principle or selfish ambition, but even in the midst of carnage, the Geneva Convention stipulates that prisoners of war should be treated with respect and not subjected to degrading punishments.

In addition, other less obviously dramatic occupations than medicine and warfare also involve life and death decisions. A local authority transport official has to decide where to place the pedestrian crossings in a busy city. The official knows, based on the last three years' statistics, that if a crossing is put in a certain place, several children's lives could probably be saved every year. Nevertheless there is a restricted budget and a need to keep the traffic flowing. These are not dissimilar conflicts from those that doctors have to face. The train driver travelling at 100 mph who sees a car suddenly stop on the level crossing in front of the train has a split second to decide whether to risk the lives of 300 people on the train by braking suddenly or whether to continue driving and kill the occupants of the car. Doctors do not usually have to make that kind of decision in peacetime.

It is interesting to note that two major ethical issues dominated the Presidential elections in the USA in 2004: the ethics of going to war in Iraq and the ethics of abortion.

PROFESSIONAL ETHICS

Clearly there is a need in many areas of activity to have an agreed ethic – an agreed code of behaviour. However, it is of special importance in those professions that have the closest, often confidential relationship with other people, such as medicine, nursing, the law and education. The aim of these 'professional ethics' is to protect the patient, client or child as well as regulating the relationship between the professionals themselves. There is an increasing requirement for professional codes of conduct to be made overt so that everybody knows what to expect. It would be difficult for patients if each doctor had a different code of ethics.

Medical ethics are there primarily to protect the patient rather than support the mystique of the profession itself.

The General Medical Council (GMC), the doctors' governing body in the UK, has issued guidelines on the duties of a doctor (Box 1.1).

Box 1.1 The duties of a doctor registered with the General Medical Council

Patients must be able to trust doctors with their lives and health. To justify that trust you must:

- Respect human rights
- Make the care of your patient your first concern
- Provide a good standard of practice and care
- Recognize and work within your professional competence
- Keep your professional knowledge and skills up to date
- Co-operate with colleagues
- Protect and promote the health of patients and the public
- Act without delay if you have good reason to believe that you or a colleague is not fit to practise
- Make efficient use of the resources available to you
- Respect each patient's dignity and individuality
- Treat every patient politely and considerately
- Respect your patient's privacy and maintain confidentiality
- Make sure your personal beliefs do not adversely affect patient care
- Work with patients as partners in their care
- Listen to patients
- Give patients the information they want or need in a way they can understand
- Respect patient's rights to reach decisions with you about their treatment and care
- Obtain informed consent where appropriate
- Be honest and trustworthy
- Never discriminate unfairly against patients or colleagues
- Act with integrity
- Be open with patients especially if something goes wrong
- Never abuse your position as a doctor
- Never act in ways which undermine public confidence in the medical profession.

You are personally accountable for your professional practice and must always be prepared to justify your actions and decisions.

HOW DOES THIS AFFECT THE INDIVIDUAL DOCTOR?

It is the responsibility of all medical students to think carefully about the moral basis for medical practice (see Chapter 4), and to analyse how this fits with their future career. We shall never know Dr Harold Shipman's motives and morals when he started medicine but certainly, later on, other motives overcame the ethical obligation of not harming patients. Whether a consensus is still possible in a pluralistic society will be discussed in Chapter 5. We will also outline how an individual doctor should act if he or she disagrees with the general view of the ethics of a given situation and how 'conscience clauses' can work (Chapters 5 and 6).

THE SCOPE OF MEDICAL ETHICS

Once people are become exposed to medical ethics, they can become overenthusiastic and find ethical dilemmas in every bed! Many everyday treatment decisions are straightforward for the doctor and based on simple scientific knowledge (i.e. they are technical, not ethical). For example, if a patient has clear evidence of a ruptured aortic aneurysm, the right plan of treatment is to operate urgently. An ethical dilemma arises if the patient has some additional co-morbidity that makes the anaesthetic particularly risky. Otherwise, the benefit of operating outweighs the risk of not doing so (see Chapter 12). To take another example, the choice of antibiotic to treat an infection is based on sensitivities of that particular organism to different antibiotics. An ethical dilemma arises either if the side-effects could be worse than the infection (which is rare) or if the antibiotic is very expensive and its use would deprive others of care or if there is a limited supply and patients have to be prioritized by severity of infection or some other criteria. If, on the other hand, the antibiotic is not really necessary, its use could encourage bacterial resistance and reduce its future effectiveness in patients.

When the subject of medical ethics is raised, many people think immediately of extreme treatments such as face transplants, cybertechnology or new techniques for cloning their favourite sporting idol. The media love to highlight these dramatic new developments but, although they are exciting, they will probably ultimately affect a relatively small number of people and have little relevance to the routine practice of medicine today. Everyday medical ethics include important but apparently mundane matters such as telling patients the truth, not gossiping about their confidential details in the hospital lift, respecting their right to take decisions about their own illnesses, and not operating on them without their consent (except under special circumstances).

One issue currently dominating the UK National Health Service is the rationing of treatments and attempts to ensure equity of access. No country in the world, however rich, will ever be able to afford every treatment its people would wish, and prioritization (which sounds more acceptable than rationing!) will always be necessary. The problem is how to prioritize fairly and by criteria that are generally acceptable to patients and professionals. This will be discussed in more detail in Chapter 10.

LEARNING MEDICAL ETHICS: WHERE TO START

The subject of medical ethics is now included in all medical school curricula, although the format and the stage in the course at which it is introduced varies greatly. The situation is much better than in the middle of the twentieth century when students were just supposed to assimilate ethics by watching their teachers (some good and some bad) and if they were lucky they had one lecture on medical ethics, the main point of which was to deter doctors from sleeping with their patients! Many students these days feel burdened with problems posed by ethics that have no apparent solutions. As a result, the temptation is to abandon the effort and hope that instinct and inspiration comes to the rescue at the right time. Medical decisions are too important for that, however. The purpose of this book is to make sense of the apparent confusion, and to give you the map that helps to lead you out of the maze.

Curriculum

In 1998 teachers of ethics and law in UK medical schools met together and produced a consensus statement on what should be covered (Consensus Statement, 1998). They concluded that the goal should be to create good doctors who will enhance and protect the health and medical welfare of the people they serve in ways that fairly and justly respect their dignity, autonomy and rights. Four key components were identified:

- To understand the values that underpin the practice of good medicine, to reflect on one's own beliefs and appreciate alternative and sometimes competing approaches.
- To be able to think critically about ethical issues and analyse the ethical components of different types of medical decisions while being aware of one's emotional reactions.
- To be aware of the main professional obligations on UK doctors, especially those specified by the GMC as well as the main international Codes and Declarations.
- To understand that ethical principles are integral components, not only of extraordinary situations but in everyday medicine and to learn to apply the principles in practice.

They recommended that these should be brought about by a 'balanced, sustained, academically rigorous, and clinically relevant presentation of both ethics and law and the relationship and tensions between them'. Ethics needs to be a core subject throughout the curriculum and be seen to be important rather than relegated to those few corners left by apparently more important subjects. It must be compulsory, as it is quite unfair for a student to qualify and then be under the watchful eye of the GMC without knowing what standards are required. However, many medical schools give opportunities for those who want to pursue the subject further, to undertake ethics projects in elective time or undertake an intercalated BSc or B.Med.Sci degree.

CONCLUSION

Consideration of medical ethics often appears to create more questions than answers. We are convinced that there are answers, and a large amount of consensus can be achieved. There are many books containing in-depth discussion of ethical issues and there are several journals devoted to the subject. This book is designed to give clear practical guidance and a sense of perspective, by focusing on key ethical areas, and to act as a stimulus to critical thinking. It also challenges the reader to adopt a clear value system; finally, it aims to instil something of the excitement and interest in a subject that will never disappear but, instead, become more and more relevant with every new medical development and every step of each doctor's career.

Summary
- Medical ethics are the obligations of a moral nature that govern the practice of medicine.
- They are concerned with the everyday care of patients as well as research and new and exciting treatments and an ethical framework needs to be brought to the practice of medicine from outside.
- Other professions and occupations also have difficult ethical decisions – medicine is not unique.
- The challenge to the medical profession is to find common ground for an agreed body of professional ethics.
- The subject of medical ethics is not an 'optional extra' to medical studies.
- All potential doctors must be aware of the present ethical framework given by the General Medical Council and other medical bodies.

MYTHS AND MISUNDERSTANDINGS

Before we look into medical ethics in more detail, it is important to clear away some of the many misunderstandings that cloud ethical discussion. When debating such issues people often quote catch phrases that are passed on without analysis and which, although they sound helpful, may in practice inhibit clear thinking. We have selected 10 common examples and discuss them below.

1. 'CONFUSING COMPARISONS'

The most common mistake in any discussion, public or private, is to lump together issues that are not really the same and to argue at cross-purposes. Definitions and the exact details of a clinical situation are important. For example, the following actions have all been labelled 'euthanasia' or 'mercy killing', yet each has different ethical perspectives and needs to be analysed separately:

- Turning off the respirator when a patient is brain dead.
- Withdrawing a treatment that is no longer of benefit.
- Withholding a treatment that may be futile.
- Physician-assisted suicide.

● Euthanasia of patients without their consent.
● Ending patients' lives against their will.

When analysing the ethics of any clinical decision the first step is to define the issues and clarify the distinctions (see Chapters 13 and 14). The General Medical Council (GMC, 2002) has given guidance on withdrawing and withholding life-prolonging treatments.

2. 'MEDICINE CAN PRODUCE ITS OWN ETHICS'

The implication of this widely held view is that medicine does not need any outside control or interference because any new treatment we discover or devise must be good for the patient. This is, of course, completely false. Medical science is ethically neutral and, like nuclear energy, can be used for good or harm. Nuclear energy itself does not dictate whether it is used to cure cancer or make an atomic bomb.

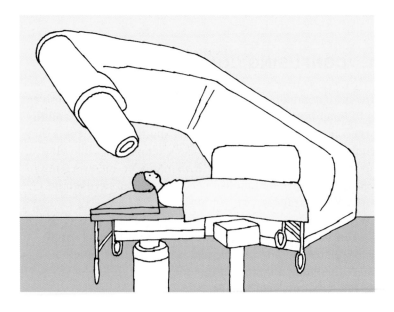

Just because we have (fortunately) become used to medical science being used to help and heal, we must not be lulled into a sense of false security. Not very long ago in Europe, under Hitler, medical skills were used to harm and destroy. This still occurs in a number of countries today. Even when we are trying to benefit the patient we have to ask the question not '**can** it be done'? but '**should** it be done'? Moreover, the more powerful a drug or the more complex a surgical or psychiatric intervention, the more potential there is for harm as well as good. Therefore, although we may intend to do good we might actually do harm and the harm (e.g. death) may be far worse than the intended good. This is why patients and doctors need to know the risks of a treatment so that consent is truly informed. Treatment plans and clinical research designs all aim to maximize the good and reduce the risk of harm. Risk/benefit analysis is a practical way of helping such decisions. Ethical principles such as autonomy (Chapter 7), beneficence (Chapter 8) and justice (Chapter 10) must be applied to medicine to control and direct it to the benefit of all.

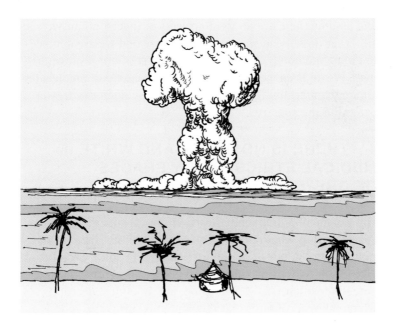

3. 'THERE IS ONLY ONE RIGHT ANSWER TO AN ETHICAL DILEMMA'

Some people treat ethical questions like crossword puzzles: given a clue, they debate and agonize while trying to find the one answer that exactly fits the spaces in the grid. The answer to a newspaper crossword puzzle can be discovered the next day, but it may take months or even years before we know whether a clinical decision was right! Sometimes, there is a generally agreed correct answer, but two doctors with exactly the same set of values may make different decisions for an individual patient because they give different weights to the same values. This is discussed in detail with clinical examples in Chapter 12. Obviously we should all strive for the ideal answer but the very fact there is a dilemma is because the situation is not always ideal, and we cannot always please everyone or do good without risk of harm. This can easily make us feel like failures if we cannot find easy solutions.

On the other hand it is possible to swing to the other extreme and assume there are no right answers or indeed no answers at all – that there is no way out of the maze and we are doomed to go up and down blind paths for the rest of our professional lives. We do need answers, and endless discussions and debates, although entertaining, do not help the busy doctor to treat a patient in the surgery.

4. 'THERE IS NO BLACK AND WHITE IN MEDICAL ETHICS – ONLY SHADES OF GREY'

This comment is frequently heard. It sounds superficially attractive, but what does it mean? It implies that there is no right or wrong, but only right decisions with some wrong or vice versa. As we have mentioned above, all treatments have potential for harm as well as good, but an ethical decision which takes account of that fact and maximizes the good is a right decision. A consent form for clinical research that protects the autonomy of patient or volunteer is right even if some unexpected side-effect occurs. We will be discussing in Chapter 4 how we define what is right or wrong, while Chapter 12 analyses how giving priority to one principle over another in a given situation avoids the greyness of trying to merge competing principles.

5. 'RELIGION SHOULD BE KEPT OUT OF THE DISCUSSION OF MEDICAL ETHICS'

It is a strange notion that those doctors with a religious faith are biased whereas those without are neutral. A non-religious philosophy also contains equally strong personal values: it is just as biased. We all bring our own value systems into the practice of medicine. A Buddhist doctor who gives a very high value to all sentient life has just as valid a view as a secular utilitarian who values a foetus no more than a gallbladder.

> For an atheist to call a Christian 'biased' is like a Cornishman accusing a Yorkshireman of speaking English with an accent!

However, there is a duty on all of us to be transparent about the basis of our values, whether religious or secular, and to explain them with integrity. It is even more important to explore the logical consequences of each value system, if applied consistently to the practice of medicine. We will be doing this in Chapter 4. Doctors who say they believe that humans are merely naked apes – with no more intrinsic value than animals – do not actually practise on that assumption when it comes to caring for their patients. On the other hand, those whose religion teaches great respect for animal life because of a belief in the reincarnation of souls into animals will be reluctant to kill rats even if they are devouring the grain stores or bringing disease to humans.

A newspaper survey published in the *Daily Telegraph* (27 December 2004) found that 44 per cent of people in the UK believe in God and the majority of the remainder are not sure. The proportion of 'believers' may be higher amongst doctors. If religion is kept out of medical ethics, the values of many doctors and patients will be ignored. The importance of the spiritual dimension of patient care has become increasingly recognized in recent years (Culliford, 2002; Royal College of Psychiatrists, 2005).

6. 'DOCTORS' PERSONAL BELIEFS SHOULD NOT AFFECT THE MEDICINE THEY PRACTISE'

According to the General Medical Council guidelines doctors should make sure their 'personal beliefs do not **adversely** affect patient care'. There are two ways in which the word 'belief' can be understood in this context: First, a doctor may have a personal belief in a certain treatment – a treatment that is not standard or evidence-based. For example, some years ago, we came across a doctor who believed that a teaspoon of petroleum jelly taken after each meal would heal duodenal ulcers! Patients kept up this unpleasant treatment for many years but eventually needed conventional treatment for their ulcers. This 'belief' denied the patients an effective treatment and put them at risk of a perforation or bleed. Having said that, we must be careful not to condemn all unorthodox treatments out of hand. History shows that what started as a 'wild idea' sometimes turns out to be a breakthrough. Whoever would have approved of the old tradition of putting mouldy bread on a wound until penicillin was discovered from such a mould? The important point about these 'beliefs' is that they can be tested by the scientific method and patients are protected from most adverse effects by being treated under carefully controlled conditions.

The second type of 'belief' is in the religious or non-religious value systems referred to in the previous section and discussed in Chapter 4, which inform doctors' personal ethics. Some ethicists feel that private and public ethics should be separated and that a doctor should be forced to do what the patient requests, if it is legal, and should not be allowed the luxury of a conscience clause. To forbid doctors to allow these basic beliefs to affect the practice of medicine is to destroy their integrity as people and make them the slave of 'a system'. After all, another of the GMC duties of a doctor is 'to act with integrity'.

In practice there may be only a few occasions when a doctor finds that the requested treatment goes against a deeply held belief; moreover what the doctor believes may, in the long run, be for the patient's good. Abortion is the commonest example and integrity demands that doctors give a clear, non-threatening explanation to a patient of why they could not recommend an abortion on conscience grounds. As the GMC guidelines recommend, they should also inform the patient of her right to a second opinion (GMC, 2001). (The recommendation that the doctor should refer the patient to a colleague who they know will agree to the patient's wishes may breach the doctor's human rights. This is currently under discussion.) This doctor could be an excellent general practitioner or even an obstetrician and gynaecologist. Chapters 5 and 6 discuss conscience clauses in legislation.

However, a doctor with a strong ethical objection to all animal experiments cannot in all conscience prescribe any of the current drugs, all of which have to go through animal testing to be licensed. This would probably be deemed to affect patient care adversely and although the doctor could refer to colleagues every time a prescription was needed, this would be incompatible with the practice of modern medicine.

Alternative and complementary systems of care often combine these two different types of belief. They are usually based on a religious philosophy (e.g. yoga, acupuncture, aromatherapy and reflexology), but do not on the whole have a strong scientific evidence base. Many people using them are unaware of the philosophies underlying them.

7. 'ETHICS SHOULD BE LEFT TO THE EXPERTS'

It is quite understandable that busy doctors do not want to be involved in analysis and discussions of every clinical decision. They just want simple rules to go by which avoid too much thought and want 'experts' to make the decisions for them. The experts may be lawyers, philosophers or academic ethicists. The tragedy of the present situation is that ethical standards are being enforced, and sometimes defined, as a result of litigation. The fear of litigation is leading to overinvestigation and treatment which may not be in the patient's best interest and sometimes it prevents doctors from doing good. It is sad that 2000 years after Jesus Christ told the familiar Parable of the Good Samaritan – where a despised member of a different race helped a man mugged and left for dead at the roadside – the USA has had to introduce 'Samaritan laws' to protect doctors from litigation. These laws protect a doctor who goes to the aid of an accident victim at the roadside if the victim subsequently fails to recover fully. The place of law is discussed in Chapter 6.

Philosophers are experts in framing questions, logic and reasoning, but the personal moral opinion of a professor of philosophy carries no more authority than that of a first-year medical student. Mclean (1993) rejects the authority of philosophy to give guidance on moral matters and questions the whole direction of the present bioethics enterprise.

> *All these philosophers do is disguise the answer they want to give – that is to say, their own moral opinions – as the verdict of philosophical enquiry.*
> (Mclean, 1993, page 17)

An increasing number of philosophers and ethicists are specializing full time in the identification, analysis and solution of the problems that doctors face, but some of them have had little practical experience of everyday difficult clinical problems, and to a busy doctor they can seem remote. In North America many hospitals these days have full-time clinical ethicists who have been trained specifically in clinical situations, some of whom come from a medical background; indeed in some institutions an ethicist is available 24 hours a day. They can build up a wealth of experience of different clinical situations and the ways they have been resolved in the past or in other institutions.

In the UK, hospital trusts are beginning to set up clinical ethics committees, which are useful for drafting hospital policies and guidelines but not much help with an acute clinical problem in the middle of the night. A closer link between academic ethicists and practising doctors would benefit both, but ultimately medical ethics needs to be developed by doctors and not merely left as an academic pursuit.

8. 'EMOTION SHOULD BE KEPT OUT OF ETHICAL DISCUSSIONS'

One does not have to be involved in field of medicine for very long before realizing the strong emotions that clinical decisions engender. A typical radio or TV ethical debate often generates more heat than light. What then is the place of emotions in making clinical decisions or defining ethics? On the one hand they cannot be ignored, but on the other hand the concept 'because I **feel** it is right, it **is** right' is a shaky basis for a professional ethic. The argument between reason and emotion as a basis for moral behaviour goes back to the views of the philosophers David Hume and Immanuel Kant in the eighteenth century: Hume asserted that morality depends on fundamental aspects of human nature such as self-interest and altruistic sympathy whereas Kant talked about ideas that are imposed on the senses and are logically prior (a priori) to the materials they relate to. It is certainly a myth that a doctor can avoid the emotional tension of making difficult decisions or conveying difficult facts to patients. A doctor who can tell a patient that he or she has inoperable cancer without finding it emotionally draining has lost all sensitivity and compassion.

It is possible for someone's ethics to be determined by these feelings to an unacceptable degree. For example, for a large part of the twentieth century, doctors commonly told direct lies or used misleading euphemisms for cancer, to avoid the embarrassment of having to discuss life and death issues. Another example is when a member of the ward staff calls the crash team to a patient because 'she was such a nice lady', even though a decision has been made not to attempt resuscitation. Feelings about patients in certain situations are not necessarily wrong but they must be identified and brought into the open. If doctors start to initiate treatment because they particularly like a patient then, by the same token, they may fail to take the correct action because of a dislike.

Many medical treatments – not just surgical operations – involve considerable pain and discomfort during the course of healing. If emotion dictates the treatment, then a chance of cure might be missed. This is particularly true of treating children and is also why the GMC recommend that doctors do not treat members of their own family or close friends. Balanced emotions can be a strong motive for good care; uncontrolled emotions can lead to unethical practice.

9. 'A DOCTOR CANNOT REFUSE A PATIENT'S REQUEST FOR TREATMENT'

Over the last 50 years the focus of a consultation has swung from the opinions of the patronizing doctor to the wishes and rights of the patient. No longer do patients come with symptoms for diagnosis and advice, but with a self-made diagnosis demanding a specific treatment (often waving a long print-out from the Internet!). This is, of course, a gross overgeneralization, but it does reflect the trend. The issue of a patient's autonomy, which some ethicists think is the paramount ethical principle, will be considered in detail in Chapter 7. But here we will discuss whether or not there are circumstances in which a doctor can legitimately and ethically refuse the patient's request for treatment.

One example is when the treatment would be futile – that is it would produce no benefit at the cost of pain, discomfort or risk. This often arises in the context of palliative care for dying patients. They, or more often their relatives, push for 'everything to be done' including giving another course of radiotherapy, chemotherapy or even surgery which will give further discomfort, or nausea and vomiting, with no chance of significant improvement. Sometimes a brief physical improvement may be achievable but with a large psychological risk. It is tempting for doctors to agree to such treatments for the sake of the relatives or to make themselves feel better because 'they are doing something', even though they really know it is of no benefit. In the USA such pressure has become so strong that staff in some hospitals have issued a formal statement that 'they will not undertake futile treatments'.

Second, doctors may refuse a treatment because they believe it is not in the patient's best interest because the risks outweigh the benefits. The patient may argue that he or she wants the treatment and is prepared to take the risk. This does not absolve the doctor from giving the best advice possible but, as always, the patient has a right to consult another doctor who may see the risks differently. Inevitably there are stories of patients going from doctor to doctor until they at last find someone who agrees to the treatment – sometimes with disastrous results.

Some patients who have been refused an operation use the ultimate attempt at persuasion by asking whether a surgeon will 'do the operation privately'! The wise surgeon will have the same criteria and give the same advice and treatment in private practice as in the NHS.

Third, a doctor may refuse treatment because, although it may not be harmful to the individual patient, it puts other patients at risk. A good example of this is a request for antibiotics for an uncomplicated upper respiratory tract infection – a common request to GPs. Antibiotics have very little effect but frequent prescribing has led to increased bacterial resistance, which may endanger patients in the future when serious infections will not respond. The Standing Medical Advisory Committee was so concerned about this that its document *The Path of Least Resistance* advised GPs not to prescribe antibiotics in this situation and also to restrict the length of antibiotic use in other mild infections (Standing Medical Advisory Committee, 1996).

Fourth, a doctor may refuse to give an expensive treatment when a cheaper one is just as good for that illness. Again, antibiotics illustrate this principle as do analgesics. Patients may request the latest expensive drug when trials have shown there is little difference between it and the standard treatment. The National Institute for Health and Clinical Excellence (NICE) was set up in England and Wales to provide information for such decisions. Sometimes the more expensive drug acts more quickly even if not more effectively so it may have other advantages. This leads us to the final myth or misunderstanding.

10. 'IT IS UNETHICAL FOR A TREATMENT TO BE WITHHELD BECAUSE OF LACK OF MONEY'

If only! Financing health is one of the most contentious and far reaching discussions not only in the West but throughout the world. The NHS was set up so that patients are not prevented from access to care because of lack of money. Health care is 'free at the point of delivery'. But it has to be paid for somehow. In the UK it is financed from taxation, whereas in other countries it is by private or state insurance schemes. In many countries, however, some or all of the payment is requested from the patient at the time of treatment and, if patients cannot pay, they may not be treated. No country in the world, however rich, can possibly finance for everybody the care they need, let alone the care they wish. With the huge cost of many drugs and interventions, some have to be rationed and priorities have to be determined, otherwise patients with less severe illnesses will take all the money from those with greater needs. The ethical dilemma, if the principle of justice is accepted, is how and on what criteria the prioritization should be made. This is discussed in detail in Chapter 10.

The next chapter explores the different ways of devising ethical guidance on these and many other issues.

Summary

- Issues that are ethically different may appear to be similar.
- Medical science cannot produce its own ethics.
- There is not always only one right answer to a dilemma.
- There can be clear, right answers not just shades of grey.
- Religion is just as valid as secular philosophies in ethical discussions.
- Doctors must be careful how their personal beliefs impact on their practice and must be transparent about it. Scientific beliefs can be tested.
- Emotion is an important influence on ethical decisions but must be recognized and identified.
- Medical ethics cannot just be left to experts; doctors must be involved.
- A doctor may refuse a patient's request for treatment in certain circumstances.
- Financial factors cannot be left out of ethical decisions.

HOW CAN ETHICAL GUIDANCE BE FOUND?

ETHICAL THEORIES

We have already explored some of the problems, analysed some of the issues, and dispelled some of the confusion. But how can we make sense of medical ethics by developing a consistent logical system of thought that can produce practical guidelines, and how can we decide what is right or wrong? We need a way of testing an action against some criteria – we need ethical theories. These theories are then informed by values to produce ethical principles from which everyday rules can be derived (Figure 3.1). Values will be discussed in Chapter 4 and each of the main principles in Chapters 7–11.

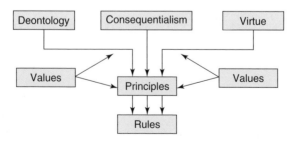

Figure 3.1 Ethical theories

There are three ways we can obtain ethical guidance. These in turn give rise to three established ethical theories:

1. We can see how a particular the action compares with a set of preordained obligations and duties and check whether these are right or wrong. This is deontological ethics (from the Greek *deon*, meaning 'duty').
2. We can anticipate the likely results of an action and decide whether it is beneficial or harmful. This is consequentialist (teleological) ethics.
3. We can ask what virtues a well-motivated person would do in the circumstances, because virtuous people tend to do good and right things. This is virtue ethics.

Let us illustrate these three approaches with an everyday example: Why should a surgeon obtain consent from a patient for a straightforward necessary operation? The deontologist says it is because the doctor has a duty to respect the patient's autonomy (right to choose). The consequentialist argues that if consent is not obtained, the patient may later wish he or she had not agreed to the operation and claim to be unaware of the side-effects. Moreover the patient might even turn round and sue the surgeon – definitely a bad consequence for the surgeon! The virtue ethicist would explain the virtues of compassion, integrity and conscientiousness that motivates the surgeon to discuss the operation in detail and obtain consent. They all agree that obtaining consent is good and right but for different reasons and it is the intention of all to do the patient good and not harm.

We will now look at the three theories in more detail:

DEONTOLOGY – DUTY-BASED ETHICS

This theory emphasizes obligations on the doctor based upon good, universal, moral principles, even if the consequences may sometimes be harmful or the intentions dubious. The extreme form of this approach is 'the categorical imperative' associated

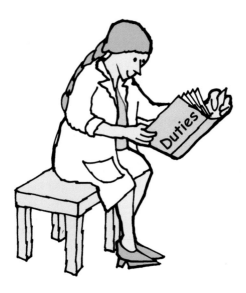

with the work of Immanuel Kant (1724–1804). This puts the principle of duty as supreme, i.e. we should only act in conformity with what we understand to be a moral law. Right actions flow from right principles and these principles are universal, not just for us in a particular situation. Deontology has several subdivisions, as illustrated in Figure 3.2.

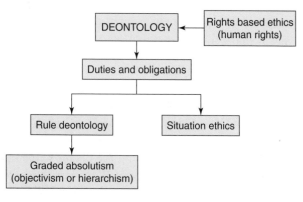

Figure 3.2 Subdivisions of deontology

Rights-based ethics

Some writers refer to patients' rights or liberal individualism as a separate theory, but it is also evident that doctors' obligations arise from patients' legitimate rights. In the example above on conformed consent, the doctor's obligation to ask for consent arises from the patient's right as a human being to exercise autonomy – to have some say on what happens to his or her own body. Sadly, the common experience today of people campaigning for their rights is often because others have neglected their duty and obligations. So rights and obligations are not necessarily competing but may be two sides of the same coin. The principles that most ethicists pick out as being the most important to medicine are: autonomy, beneficence (and non-maleficence), justice and fairness, truth and integrity. These can be described in terms of either the **obligations** for the doctor or the **rights** of the patient. Truth telling can be seen both as a fundamental duty of the doctor and as the patient's right to be given correct information and not be misled.

Rule deontology

Rule deontology is a branch of deontology in which a moral act is compared with a set of rules or moral principles to determine whether it is right or wrong, ethical or unethical. Rule deontology is about correct reasoning, not feelings. To caricature the approach, the moral law obliges me to give money to the poor but that does not mean I have to like them!

For example, the commandments that God gave to Moses in the thirteenth century BC – the Ten Commandments – give 10 general universal rules of conduct which can be applied to many aspects of human behaviour, some being more specific than others. There are eight negative prohibitions and two positive commands (Exodus 20). For example 'You shall not murder' and 'You shall not steal' have wide acceptance as principles against which people's actions can be judged as right and wrong. Of relevance to doctors involved in giving evidence in court is 'Do not give false testimony against your neighbour', which is still the basis of the severe punishments for perjury in British courts. These prohibitions are treated very seriously even though you could argue that on rare occasions, many people might benefit from a person being murdered or a thief stealing somebody's money and giving it to the poor.

Absolutism

Some deontologists go so far as to say there are some principles that are absolute and can never be overridden under any circumstances. For example, 'You shall not kill' means there are no circumstances in which killing would be right – even for the police to kill a terrorist who is about to blow up a train containing 300 people. They would say there are no circumstances in which a lie is justified, even to save the lives of innocent people. It is interesting that the Jews to whom the commandment 'You shall not kill' was given were permitted the death penalty for serious crimes. Even though you may not go the whole way with the absolutists, it is worth asking if there are any acts that are always wrong whatever the circumstance. Two possible candidates are torture for fun and rape. Whereas some people might justify limited torture in occasional situations in order to obtain information that would save innocent lives, it is difficult ever to justify torture for fun and rape.

Graded absolutism

This is also known as objectivism or hierarchism. Most deontologists accept a graded absolutism, which means that there is a series of moral laws which can act as absolutes in isolation but occasionally another law or principle may have to override it. In other words there is a hierarchy of absolute moral laws and those higher up in the hierarchy may occasionally have priority over others lower down. The example of telling a lie to save lives in a special situation shows that the obligation of preserving life can occasionally override the obligation to tell the truth; but if it is simply inconvenient to tell the truth, convenience cannot override such an important principle. A person may be freed from the obligations of a moral duty by obeying a higher one, but there are no right acts outside the moral law. Many illustrations of graded absolutism (hierarchism) are given in Chapter 12.

Situation ethics

There are two different ways in which the word 'situation' is used in medical ethics. The first is the idea that general rules must be applied in particular situations and, as we have seen, may be given different weightings. Unapplied moral principles are of no help in medical practice but this does not mean the situation itself produces its own ethics (see Subjective individual ethics, below). Secondly, the term situation ethics was coined in the 1960s by Joseph Fletcher, a Christian theologian in the USA, and is, surprisingly, a specific form of deontology. He believes in absolute moral laws but that in practice there is only one – love. He takes this from the teaching of Jesus Christ and his followers which emphasized love for others as the basis of moral behaviour. In particular he points to Jesus' declaration that the Old Testament Law, such as the 10 commandments, is summarized in just two: first, 'Love God' and second, 'Love your neighbour as yourself' (Luke 10: 27). Therefore, Fletcher argues that love overrides any other moral laws and the question to ask about a decision is not 'is it right?' but 'is it loving?' (Fletcher, 1966).

Applied to the practice of medicine this is often a good question but, to take an extreme example, if a male doctor decides that the most loving thing to do for his patient is to make love to her because she is lonely and unloved, the situational ethicist suggests that the act is right and good and overrides any abstract law such as 'Do not commit adultery'. The problem with this approach is that it becomes very subjective, and we can easily deceive ourselves and there are often several other people involved. The doctor's wife might not consider that adultery with a patient was the most loving thing to do! It is also based on the misunderstanding that laws and love are incompatible. Whereas altruistic love is a fundamental part of virtue ethics (see Chapter 16), Fletcher's situation ethics is not a sound basis for medical practice.

CONSEQUENTIALISM (TELEOLOGY)

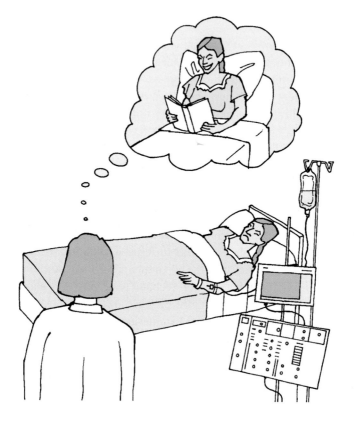

Consequentialists reject the idea that universal moral laws can be brought to a decision. The only way to find out if a decision or action is right or wrong, they argue, is to look at the consequences. One problem is that it may be possible to see the short-term consequences but very difficult to anticipate the long-term results. The purest form of this theory is utilitarianism, which is associated with the eighteenth- and nineteenth-century philosophers David Hume (1711–1776), John Stewart Mill (1806–1873) and Jeremy Bentham (1748–1832) of University College, London, who rejected worn-out deontological moral rules in favour of reform and of a commendable attempt to lift moral burdens from the poor.

Utilitarianism

Utilitarianism states that a moral act is one which brings the greatest balance of good over evil for the greatest number of people. This naturally leads to expediency and inconsistency. So, for example, if a doctor makes a serious, culpable mistake in the treatment of a patient, if the greater good of many other patients would be served by ignoring it instead of exposing it and possibly punishing the doctor, utilitarians might consider this the right thing to do. One could argue that it would shake the confidence of many patients if they knew what had happened and if the doctor were suspended, treatment for many others would be delayed. This argument was recently used successfully when the High Court overruled the General Medical Council (GMC) suspension of a plastic surgeon on the grounds of an affair with a married patient. Deontologists, by contrast, would argue that the doctor seriously failed his duty of care to the patient and therefore should be punished whatever the consequences.

Jeremy Bentham produced a scoring system called the hedonistic calculus. For him, pleasure was the 'good' and pain the 'evil'. Therefore a score could be given to the seven aspects of each, such as intensity and duration, and the pain score then subtracted from the pleasure score (Bentham, 1789/1961). The units were 'hedons'! As we know, pleasure and pain are very subjective and it is difficult to compare one person's pleasure with another's, or one pleasure with another. For a patient, is the pleasure of taking a few first steps after a spinal injury, although somewhat painful, greater or less than the pleasure of lying in bed pain-free and eating a nice meal?

John Stewart Mill classified pleasures as higher order, which included intellectual, cultural, creative and spiritual pleasures, or lower order (elementary) pleasures such as eating, drinking, resting and sex (Mill, 1861/1998). We will discuss ways of measuring quality of life with objective criteria in Chapters 4 and 10.

Utilitarianism also involves the principle that 'the end justifies the means'. If the aim to bring as much pleasure to as many people as possible is good, then any means can be used to accomplish it, even if they contradict the deontologist's moral principles. One could justify painful and even dangerous research on a few people if it brought some benefit to many; so in that case the principle of individual autonomy can be ignored. Pure utilitarianism eliminates the essential ingredients of moral thinking.

VIRTUE ETHICS

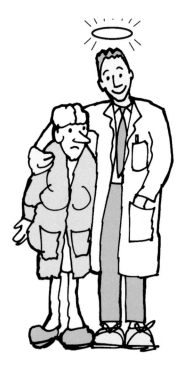

The virtue ethicists observe that many of the moral rules and duties are negative and ignore important aspects of relationships and motivation. Rather than make binding rules and duties, they argue, we should concentrate on changing people's attitudes and character, and they will then want to do the right thing. Is the doctor who gets up at night to treat a patient with an acute illness through compassion and concern, better than one who does the same thing from a sense of duty? Is the person who cares because they are paid, worse than the person who cares for long hours without receiving a penny? Virtue ethics has been the subject of debate for many of the great moral teachers of the past but has been revived in the last 50 years by philosophers such as Elizabeth Anscombe (1919–2001), Alasdair MacIntyre (b. 1929) and Richard Taylor (1919–2003) (Anscombe, 1958; MacIntyre, 1981; Taylor, 1985).

Some of the virtues that are needed for ethical practice are:

- Compassion
- Discernment
- Trustworthiness
- Integrity
- Conscientiousness
- Good relationships.

Being conscientious and discerning, however, does not mean a person is conscientious about the right things. Courage is not necessarily an ethical virtue because someone can be courageous in rescuing a drowning person from the sea but presumably, a suicide bomber also needs courage. Rules without the right motivation can become burdens that exclude any feeling, while virtues without a framework can become subjective and unfocused. As in many walks of life the pendulum swings from one extreme to the other instead of oscillating gently around a balanced centre. Chapter 16 deals with the personal qualities required for a good ethical doctor but we are not automatically paragons of virtue!

SUBJECTIVE INDIVIDUAL ETHICS

There are a number of other approaches to ethics that rely more on the individual than on ethical theories. These ethical non-theories comprise a group of philosophies in which the basis of decisions is not derived from a system of thought that can be discussed or agreed upon with other people.

Relativism

According to relativism there is no objective right or wrong but only right or wrong as each person sees it. In other words, my view of whether a medical decision is right may be different from yours, not because we disagree on the application of principles to a given situation, but because we are coming from different viewpoints. You cannot say that I am wrong and I cannot say that you are right. It is interesting to observe that relativists advocate a tolerance of views except when a deontologist claims there are objective moral principles!

Post-modernism

This is a more radical form of relativism in which the question is no longer 'Is it right or wrong?' but 'Is it right for me?' It is summarized by the comment 'I gave the patient this advice and it made me feel good; therefore it was right'. Post-modernism has its roots in nineteenth-century romanticism, which became popular at the end of the twentieth century. If everybody does what they happen to think is right, there can be no medical ethics and patients can have no trust in the profession as a whole. There can be no norms of behaviour in society. Of course people should have the freedom, within limits, to do things they wish, as long as other people are not affected. But society and relationships are so complex that it is very difficult to be sure someone else will not be hurt. Fortunately, few of our patients are truly alone – the great majority have family members, friends, carers, dependants or work colleagues.

Existentialism

Existentialism is based on the works of Søren Kierkegaard (1813–1855) and Jean-Paul Sartre (1905–1980). The extreme form of this view is summarized by the statement 'my choosing it makes it right'. Sartre writes 'to choose to do this or that is to affirm, at the same level, the value of what we choose; because we can never choose evil we always choose the good' (Sartre, 1947). This represents an extraordinary view of his own moral qualities. This approach is the opposite of deontological ethics and means that one cannot anticipate the rightness of a decision, because it is only in the taking of that decision that the rightness or wrongness exists. It can form no basis for discussion about medical ethics nor form the basis of a professional code of behaviour.

CONCLUSION – A SYNTHESIS

How then can we find ethical guidance? There are three main theories: deontology is duty-based, consequentialism looks at results, and virtue ethics emphasizes character. There is also a group of subjective individual ways of making ethical decisions which cannot form a basis of a professional ethic. In clinical practice we need all three theories. We need moral duties, which provide the agreed foundation of our professional ethics and from which we derive principles that are so important they can be called graded absolutes. However, when making a decision we need to look at the consequences to anticipate the effects. These can be tested, not against the hedonistic calculus of the pure utilitarian but against the same principles. For example, how do I know I am exercising beneficence if I cannot assess the effect and likely side-effects of my treatment? How can a patient exercise his or her autonomy if I do not truthfully relay the facts as far as I know them about the results of the treatment? How can I decide if a treatment is futile without anticipating its effect on that particular patient in that situation? Third, without virtue and character, care will soon become unfeeling and automatic and good principles will gradually be seen as a further burden on our practice. It has been well demonstrated that a doctor's attitude to a patient has a large therapeutic effect. We need a careful balance between cold calculating deontology and warm emotional virtue. The carrying out of duties and the calculation of consequences must be underpinned by good relationships, integrity and compassion.

Summary

- Three main ethical theories inform medical ethics.
- Deontology concentration on duties and universal moral principles.
- Consequentialism concentrates on the results of an action. Utilitarianism is its best-known form.
- Virtue ethics concentrates on a person's character.
- Subjective individualism includes relativism, post-modernism and existentialism. They cannot be used to establish a code of professional ethics.
- A balanced blend of deontology, consequentialism and virtue provides the best way of obtaining ethical guidance.

VALUES – THE MORAL BASIS OF MEDICAL ETHICS

We have described in the previous chapter various ways of thinking about ethical issues and ways in which we can derive ethical principles. But at all points in that process we have to decide what is good or bad, right or wrong and what is the value of the different patients we are treating and the good we are trying to do them. Politicians love to talk about 'family values' without attempting to define them. Do they mean the strict paternalist regime of a Victorian middle-class family or a modern lesbian couple bringing up a small boy? The task of ethics is to try to develop a normative theory of value because value is at the heart of moral theory, which in turn leads to the ethical principles that govern our actions.

VALUE

The word 'value' has several different meanings which need clarification. First, it can be objective or subjective:

● Objective values are those that are considered good and therefore should be sought after (e.g. justice and health).

● Subjective values, on the other hand, are things that people desire and therefore they become valuable (e.g. pleasure and wealth).

Diamonds, for example, can be considered as both: on the one hand, they are enduring and beautiful, but on the other hand, their value goes up because so many people want them.

Second, value can be intrinsic or instrumental:

● Intrinsic or inherent value is applied to things that are good in themselves, such as life, health, freedom from pain and happiness.
● Instrumental value refers to those things that are the means of obtaining something good (but not a good way of obtaining something bad!). They are valued because they lead to something of value. For example, compassion is an instrumental value because it leads to relieving another person's distress and pain. The nine 'core values' proposed by the British Medical Association in 1995 (BMA, 1995) were: competence, caring, commitment, integrity, compassion, responsibility, confidentiality, spirit of enquiry and advocacy. These are all instrumental values promoting the intrinsic values of life, health and patient happiness. They are none the less valuable for that.

Third, value can be imparted or self-assessed (self-value):

● Imparted value is the value someone puts on another person or thing, either because they are useful to them or because they love them.
● Self-value can only apply to people and is the way people value themselves. Someone with very low self-esteem may nevertheless be highly valued by others. This is exemplified by the comment made by the relative of a 20-year-old woman who committed suicide: 'Everybody loved her but, at times, she could not love herself'.

In ancient times, Greeks and Romans were under an obligation to commit suicide when life became a burden. The reasoning that leads bioethicists John Harris, Peter Singer and others to conclude that for parents to kill their babies poses no problems for society seems to be as follows: the baby is not fully self-aware and therefore cannot value its own life (Harris, 1985; Singer, 1993, 1995). If the parents do not want it, they impart no value to it; therefore it has no value. The Christian response on the other hand, is that when Jesus publicly welcomed babies that were being kept away from him with the words 'Let the little children come to me ... for the kingdom of God belongs to such as these' (Luke 18: 16), he was imparting huge value to young children, even if they were unable (yet) fully to value themselves. (The Greek word used here *brephe*, means children under the age of two.)

To illustrate the different ideas of value further, we will step away from the emotive world of medicine and consider an everyday example.

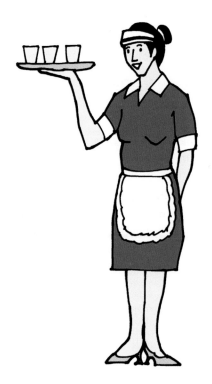

Suppose you are in a restaurant with some friends and a waitress in her early twenties comes to take your order. What is her value? There are many answers:

- She is valuable to you at the time, because you are hungry and she is going to bring you a meal (and you are going to give her a 10 per cent tip as a token of that value!).
- She is valuable to the restaurant owner (good value for money) because she is very conscientious and he only pays her £5.50 an hour.
- After talking to her you discover that she is a medical student earning extra money in the evenings. She is potentially very valuable to society because the government will not only have paid many thousands of pounds to subsidize her training but, if she subsequently becomes a full-time GP, they will rate that value at about £100 000 per year.

These three are examples of instrumental, or imparted, values. Your enjoyment of the meal could be considered an intrinsic value, albeit a subjective one, but the restaurant owner's wish to make money might not be considered to be a value at all, or, if anything, a very subjective one.

Her parents love her dearly and are very proud of her; they value her highly but the small amount they are able to give to her per month to help with her studies in no way reflects her true value to them.

These are intrinsic, imparted values; her value to them lies in her being their daughter, not in the amount they are able to pay, and is also independent of her achievements. Hopefully this value would not change, even if she failed her exams and gave up medicine.

To her new boyfriend she is potentially very valuable in terms of relation- ships and emotions and, if they stay together, she will be valuable financially, to give him the security to launch his precarious career as a musician.

This contains a mixture of intrinsic and instrumental values. His affection imparts intrinsic, objective value, but her earning potentially an instrumental value achieving a dubious sub- jective value! To everybody else she is valuable just because she is a fellow human being. This is an intrinsic, objective value.

She is just getting over 'flu and is exhausted after a hectic evening. Her student flat is cold and damp and last week she failed a biochemistry module. She feels of no use to anyone and is not sure whether she wants to continue the course.

Her self-value, both intrinsic and instrumental, is very low.

Value and quality of life

Value and quality of life are not the same, but are frequently confused. Quality of life (QoL) is measured by the patient and the observer from different objective and subjective criteria and different areas of the patient's life. The waitress described above may have a poor QoL by such tests but be very valuable to her relatives (imparted value) and may value her own life highly despite its apparent restrictions and dullness. In 2006, a High Court Judge in the case of Baby MB, on a mechanical ventilator with spinal muscular atrophy, decided that he should be kept alive because he could 'enjoy the single most important source of pleasure and emotion to a small child [subjective, intrinsic value]: his relationship with his parents and family' (instrumental value). In addition, his mother said 'Our son means the world to us' (imparted value). This is in spite of a very poor QoL judged by any objective criteria.

Value and need

Value must also be distinguished from need. If we decide to give one patient priority over another because he or she is in greater need it does not necessarily mean that we think the patient is more valuable.

Animal value

In our present society, when we value animals we consider three things: (1) their rarity, (2) their economic value and (3) their aesthetic value. Hence we put a very high value on the giant panda because it is rare, looks quaint and amuses us by its behaviour. Other animals are valued for their meat or their wool although they may not make good pets. Most people value cats more than rats because they consider them more attractive and good companions. But when we value people, why do we not use these criteria? If we did, we would logically value the rarer New Zealanders more than North Americans because there are only 3 million of them compared with 250 million! Before we send out an ambulance, we do not ask whether the patient is friendly and attractive: we mobilize all the rescue services for any person who is in trouble. This implies that, as a Western society, we function as if there is an intrinsic value to human beings, irrespective of other qualities.

VALUE SYSTEMS

Value systems are coherent groups of values that provide the basis for ethical decisions. They are derived from either religious or atheistic world-views. The religious world-views are based on revealed truth while the atheistic views rely on reasoning and observation. The 2001 Census in the UK (www. statistics.gov.uk/census2001/) asked for the first time about people's religious beliefs and the results were as follows:

Christian	71.6%
No religion	15.5%
Muslim	2.7%
Hindu	1.0%
Sikh	0.6%
Jewish	0.5%
Buddhist	0.3%

This does not mean that people necessarily **practice** the religion with which they identify but it probably means that they agree with its values even if without much conviction. The proportions may be rather different within the medical profession because over 20 per cent of doctors in the UK are of Asian origin. Many doctors probably have a mixed value system derived from several different world-views, and are deists which means they believe in a god but that he has no influence in everyday life.

RELIGIOUS WORLD-VIEWS

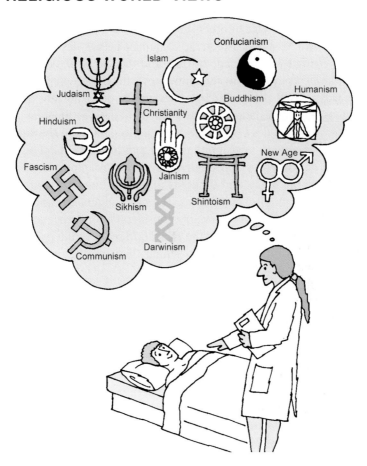

Judaism, Christianity and Islam are all monotheistic (worship one God) and refer to sacred scriptures as their authorities. They see themselves as responsible for their behaviour to God, as well as to their fellow human beings.

Judaism

This started as a formal religion about 2000 BC and the scriptures are referred to as the Tanach and are equivalent to the

Old Testament of the Christian Bible. One part of this is the Torah (teaching), which gives the laws, many in a very detailed form. Jews also refer to other religious works such as the Talmud and Mishnah. The value of human beings lies in their being created 'in the image of God' and they stress that God's will can be known as He communicates with His people in various ways. From the beginning, Jews, unlike other ancient races such as the Greeks and Romans, valued children as much as adults. Maimonedes (1135–1204) was a physician and the outstanding medieval Jewish philosopher and his 13 principles pointed out that a person's individual deeds are important to God as are the hopes and thoughts that drive him: so Judaism is not solely about obeying rules. The past judgements and advice of individual Rabbis carry considerable influence and establish 'case law'. Because the ethical principles underlying Judaism and Christianity are so similar they are often referred to as the Judaeo-Christian ethic.

Christianity

Christianity has had the major influence over the practice of medicine in the UK and much of Western Europe for 2000 years. For centuries the monasteries provided care for the sick and poor and the development of modern medicine in the eighteenth, nineteenth and twentieth centuries took place within a broad Christian culture and ethic. The scriptures are the Bible (Old and New Testaments). They teach that human beings are a distinct creation separate from other animals in their spiritual and moral make-up and are seen as God's stewards in caring for this planet. However, Christianity differs from other religions in the amazing claim that God came to this world as a man in the form of Jesus Christ who was crucified and then rose from the dead, and that this gives his teaching unique authority and affirms the high value of human beings. Forgiveness cannot be earned; it is a gift to be accepted. A summary of Jesus Christ's ethical teaching is in the Sermon on the Mount, which he illustrated by his care of the poor and outcasts of society, such as blind beggars and leprosy patients – men and women. He further stressed the importance of right motivation and described how knowing him would change attitudes and motives fundamentally.

Many Christians would also claim that God's universal moral laws, such as truth, justice, kindness are discernable by anyone from the way the world is set up (natural law) and that all human beings have an inborn sense of right and wrong (common grace).

Within Christianity, like any religion, there are different groups (denominations), some stressing certain values more than others. For example, Roman Catholics value the embryo and foetus just as highly as an adult and so are strongly anti-abortion.

Islam

Islam means 'submission to the Creator'; it was reformed by the prophet Mohammed (died AD 632) and the sacred scriptures are the Qur'an (Koran) and very detailed religious laws are contained in the Shari'a. Advice on their interpretation is given by the Masaiakh. The emphasis, as in Judaism, is obedience to laws that are commanded or forbidden by God. There is a high respect for life and Muslims are opposed to abortion and euthanasia. Many of the virtues are the same as those in the other main religions – honesty, humility, charity and kindness. In the first few centuries of Islam many of the doctors were Jews or Christians and so there was a joint influence on medical ethics. Muslims, like Christians and Jews, believe that a basic moral sense of right and wrong is part of the nature of being human – sapiental (from *Homo sapiens*). Muslims have a strong sense of fatalism (that things are ordained by God), which has an important effect on attitudes to illness and death. There are different branches of Islam with varying views.

Christianity, Judaism and Islam are all clearly deontological in their approach but also have aspects of virtue ethics (see Chapter 3).

Buddhism

Buddhism was originally founded by Buddha (the name given
to Siddhartha Gautama, 563–483 BC) in India. Buddhism has
spread to the West and there is now a Western Buddhist Order.
In contrast to the previous three religions, Buddhists do not
believe in a god, but the goal of all existence is Nirvana – 'the
complete cessation of both desire and personality' finally
attained by Buddha after many rebirths. Any sentient being –
even insects – are considered of great value and the possibility
of reincarnation into an animal is another reason for offering
animals great respect. This makes the idea of animal research
unwelcome. The six positive Dharams (precepts) are deeds of
loving kindness, open-handed generosity, stillness, simplicity
and contentment, truthful communication and transforming
ignorance into wisdom. Behaviour is far more about attitudes
than rules and fits firmly into the virtue ethics camp.

In Buddhism, Taoism and Confucianism, actions are right or
wrong, perfect or imperfect, according to the state of mind
with which they are performed; it is about psychology not
theology (Sangharaskshita, 1999) and they are accountable to
their inner conscience.

Hinduism

Hinduism is a polytheistic religion with thousands of gods and
is a synthesis of a variety of religious and cultural elements.
Each person has a spark of the universal soul. The theme of
liberation is central, and ethical actions are those that liberate
and these are seen as wealth, desire and duty, with the final
ideal being spiritual freedom (moksha). Hindus, like Buddhists,
believe in reincarnation of the soul and therefore also have a
great respect for animals – some, like the cow, being especially
sacred. They may obtain specific guidance from, and are
accountable to, their gurus.

Traditional Indian Hinduism advocates the caste system, which
is a very clear statement about the relative values of people,

from the Brahmans at the top to the 'untouchables' at the bottom. (This, however, is probably an Aryan influence rather than a religious ordering of society.) Dogma, rituals and books, such as the Vedantas, are secondary to accumulating positive karma through kind actions.

Confucianism

Confucius was born in China in 551 BC and his writings are primarily about individual morality and ethics and the proper exercise of a ruler's power. The values he proclaimed are pro-priety and etiquette, love between parents and children, right-eousness, honesty and trustworthiness, benevolence towards others and loyalty to the state.

It is important to note that many forms of alternative (comple-mentary) therapy have links with certain religions, e.g. yoga with Hinduism and acupuncture with Confucianism.

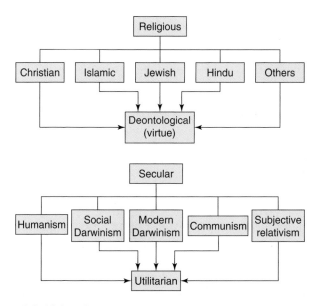

Figure 4.1 Main value systems

New Age

The New Age movement is not a unified religion and has no overall leader. It is a mixture of many different philosophies with parts derived from Eastern religions and Western Occultism and even some elements of Christianity. The overall concept is that God lies within each person and New Age practitioners look within themselves for guidance. Action by intuition leads to an absence of formal controls. Ultimately, there is no good or evil because all is one. New Age philosophy fits within the individual subjective ethics category of the previous chapter and is linked with many complementary therapies such as homeopathy, aromatherapy, etc.

NON-RELIGIOUS VALUE SYSTEMS

These systems reject any god, external revelation or written authority such as sacred scriptures, and their ethics depend on human reasoning.

Secular humanism

Secular humanism can be summed up by the statement 'moral values derive their source from human experience, ethics are autonomous and situational, needing no theological or ideological sanction' (Humanist Manifesto 2). Humanists are dedicated to human progress and, therefore, the end can justify the means, and what can be done ought to be done to this end. Leading humanist Julian Huxley saw man as 'the business manager for the cosmic process of evolution' (Huxley, 1961) (compare the Judaeo-Christian view of human beings as God's stewards). Scientific progress is seen as the agent of much of this change and humanists believe that through science humans can know the truth. Good is what improves the race and bad is what holds it back. Many humanists strongly support basic human rights and oppose racism, sexism and vast inequalities of wealth and education which stand in the way of human progress. It is clearly utilitarian in its approach (often the word humanism is confused with humanitarian or humanistic, which means seeking the welfare of human beings rather than representing a world-view). The main monotheistic religions see human beings as the culmination of a creative process – a masterpiece, albeit a damaged one, whereas to humanism they represent merely an incomplete phase of evolution. For writer John Gray, however, humanism is just a secular form of Christianity because it makes the same basic 'mistake' in thinking there is something special about the human animal (Gray, 2002).

Transhumanism

Transhumanists want to improve human beings by combining them with machines (cyborgs) (see Chapter 8 for further discussion).

Social Darwinism

Based on Darwin's theory of evolution, this philosophy, which was first annunciated by the biologist and philosopher Herbert Spencer at the end of the nineteenth century, emphasizes that the improvement of the human race is all embracing . Not only was 'the survival of the fittest' natural, it was also **morally** right. Spencer concluded that it was wrong to assist those weaker than oneself, since that would promote the survival of one who is unfit. These ideas were used to justify a eugenics programme in the USA between 1910 and 1930 and led inexorably to the Nazi programme of extermination of other races so that the leading race could survive. Followers of Social Darwinism also justified outrageous research on some people for the benefit of the 'super-race'. They confused Darwinism as a scientific theory with Social Darwinism as an ethical theory, but extrapolated from what they observed – from what is happening – to what ought to happen. This argument is known as the 'naturalistic fallacy'.

In Germany in the 1930s–1940s, a change in the underlying value system to Social Darwinism inspired by the philosopher Friedrich Nietzsche, rapidly changed caring medicinal practice into the Holocaust and brutal experimentation. Doctors were involved in this transition and a doctor, Alfred Hoche, a Professor of Medicine, was a co-author of the key book *The Destruction of Life Devoid of Value* in 1920. By the end of the Second World War 40 per cent of doctors in Germany were members of the Nazi Party (many probably being forced to join if they wanted to keep their jobs).

Social Darwinism is wholly utilitarian in its thinking, with a very limited criterion of value and is inevitably opposed to the whole health programme which is set up to care for the unfit and help them survive.

Modern Darwinism

The biologist and popular writer Richard Dawkins is one of the champions of modern Darwinist thinking. He dismisses all religious faith as an 'indulgence of irrationality' and defines faith as 'blind trust in the absence of evidence – or even in the teeth of evidence' (not a definition that many Christians would recognize) (Dawkins, 1976, page 198). However, even Dawkins admits that he needs some faith to believe that everything everywhere in the universe is the result of natural selection! He would not, of course, espouse Nazi extremism; indeed, rather than take natural selection to its logical conclusion, he states that human beings alone can rebel against our 'selfish genes'.

> There are only two types of people: those who believe dogma and know it and those who believe dogma and don't.
>
> **GK Chesterton**

Marxism/Communism

Marxism and Communism have had a huge effect on the people of the world in the last 100 years. Karl Marx (1818–1883) wanted to improve the lives of the workers who were downtrodden in a Victorian and capitalist system and it could be argued that his ideas have been distorted in practice. But communism became a system of dictatorship in which the benefit of the state was paramount, free thinking was anathema and autonomy non-existent. Class struggle constitutes the essential dynamic of society and, according to communist ethics, if the state wants to kill millions of people, that is not necessarily wrong. The only good is that which promotes the development of communism and the only bad is what hinders it: lying and slandering are justified as a means to this end. Pol Pot in Cambodia went to extremes when he announced that even people with poor eye-sight who needed to wear glasses were imperfect and therefore of less value than others who were defect free.

De-sanctifying human life

The pivotal issue in the utilitarian philosophy of people such as Peter Singer, John Harris and John Gray is the insistence that there is no intrinsic difference between humans and other ani-mals – only a difference of degree. This can lead to an eleva-tion of the value of animals or a reduction in the value of people. (Peter Singer would certainly not agree with the rea-sons given by society for valuing animals outlined on page 43.) Those who make such a distinction are guilty of 'speciesism' which, like sexism and racism, is wrong. There is nothing especially 'sacred', it is argued, about human life. In answer to the question 'What is the value of an individual human life?', Harris replies 'all we need to know is that particular individuals have their own reasons, or simply that they value their own lives. Self-awareness is the test for the person being capable of valuing it' (Harris, 1985, page 16) (we are reassured that we do not become non-persons when we are asleep!).

John Gray goes further in attacking religious and humanist ideas of morality: 'morality is a sickness peculiar to humans; the good life is a refinement of the virtues of animals. Arising from our animal natures, ethics needs no grounds; but it runs aground in the conflicts of our needs' (Gray, 2002, page 116).

Humans, he says, cannot exercise autonomy because there is no self to do the choosing.

It is beyond the scope of this book to study the behaviour of wild animals as an ethical basis for medical practice but it would make an interesting exercise!

ATTITUDES TO DEATH

For the followers of secular, atheistic philosophies, death is the end, the extinction of personality. Buddhists and Hindus look forward to rebirth and reincarnation in some form, Muslims look forward to God's judgement with uncertainty because it depends on whether they have been good enough in this life, while the Jews look to the dead re-living in the messianic age when it comes. Christians, sure of forgiveness, see death as merely the doorway to a new eternal life with God where all pain and suffering will have gone.

In a medical context it is important to realize, when looking after patients with different religious views, that after death many require very special rituals. For example, there are very detailed instructions on how a Muslim's body should be washed and shrouded. It can be very upsetting for relatives if these have been bypassed.

Let us look at two clinical scenarios and see how those committed to different world-views might react if uninhibited by a professional code of conduct.

SCENARIO 1

A 30-year-old chronic alcoholic man is admitted to hospital in hepatic failure after another drinking bout the night before. Muslims might say that as alcohol is expressly forbidden by Islamic law he has disobeyed the law and thus has experienced the just punishment for his sins; but they would still treat him kindly. Social Darwinists would say that this is just the sort of

*person we do not want to keep alive because we do not want
weak people to pass on their genes. Utilitarian humanists
might argue that if we treat him he will only go out and drink
again and so there may be no point and his general quality of
life is poor. Jews would say that although drink is not pro-
hibited, any excess of this kind is wrong but they would temper
justice with mercy and treat the patient. Christians would do
the same, pointing to Jesus' example of helping in particular
those who had fallen by the wayside. They would also want to
help him in other ways to try and stop it happening again.*

SCENARIO 2

*A baby girl is born with moderately severe Down's syndrome.
Jews, Christians and Muslims would still see her as a human
being with a spiritual nature capable of responding to God.
Buddhists and Hindus would value her life highly, just because
she is alive and would care for her. Secular utilitarians would
assess her future quality of life and decide whether or not to
look after her or let her die and they would also calculate the
long-term extra cost to the State of her care, and decide
whether it was cost effective. Some modern philosophers would
be happy for her parents to kill her, if they did not want her.
The last two groups might be dismayed that the mother did not
have an earlier screening test and then terminate the pregnancy
to prevent doctors having to make these decisions. Those with
subjective individual ethics would leave the decision to the parents based on how they felt towards the child at the time.*

CONCLUSION

These differing value systems are sometimes diametrically
opposed in their values as they impact on medical practice.
How can we possibly expect there to be a consensus and an
agreed medical ethic for the profession? This will be the subject
of the next chapter, but it is important at this stage for each

person to decide on his or her own world-view and value system and be able to answer the key question 'Why do we bother to look after sick people at all?'

Summary

- Values can be objective or subjective, intrinsic or instrumental, imparted or self-given.
- The main monotheistic religious value systems are Judaism, Christianity and Islam: these are deontological in outlook.
- Other religions – Buddhism, Hinduism, Confucianism and New Age – are more subjective.
- The main secular value systems are humanism, social Darwinism, modern Darwinism and Marxism/communism and all are utilitarian in outlook.
- There are some fundamental differences between these systems which affect attitudes to sickness, death and health care.

5

ETHICS IN CONFLICT – IS A CONSENSUS POSSIBLE?

In today's climate we all want to do 'our own thing' and not be forced to subscribe to an agreed code of rules. We want to be able to pick and choose from different philosophies and exercise the freedom to indulge in what has been dubbed 'menu morality'! But some of the philosophies in the previous chapters are dramatically opposed to each other and, of course, patients also have their own views. So doctors may disagree with doctors, and patients may disagree with doctors, and doctors and patients may both disagree with managers, lawyers and politicians.

For a profession to function consistently, and be trusted by patients, there must be recognizable and agreed standards. Indeed, as stated in Chapter 1 the main purpose of studying medical ethics is to produce general guidance for the profession as a whole. If each doctor acts independently, it will eventually destroy the profession, in the same way that cells which no longer respond to external controls become cancerous and destroy the body, and, ultimately, themselves. A caring profession needs a common morality to which all serious-minded members subscribe. The important question, however, is: How can such guidance be produced, if doctors have such different value systems?

There are several answers to this question: first, there is considerable agreement on core values between the main religions and some secular world-views. Second, most of those with more extreme views do not apply them in medical practice and are prepared to follow the general consensus. Most doctors agree that the ethical standards of behaviour with patients should be above reproach even though this standard is not always applied in other social relationships. For example, most doctors agree that committing adultery with a patient is wrong whereas some may not be quite so adamant when it comes to a friend's wife. There is general agreement that stealing from a patient is wrong whereas some doctors may not feel so strongly about stealing from the government by fiddling their tax returns! (We are **not** advocating such a double standard, but merely making an observation.)

A consensus can be reached in several ways.

1. By taking the lowest common denominator of all views.
2. By taking the majority view and allowing for exceptions (see conscience clauses).
3. By imposing a view from outside on the profession by law or governmental authority.

Taking the lowest common denominator may give a low ethical standard if only those principles that everyone agrees with are included. In a democracy a majority view will be adopted, provided the majority is substantial (e.g. at least two-thirds). It can hardly be said that it is the united view of an organization or profession if only 53 per cent agree and 47 per cent do not. However, it is quite possible for Parliament to enact a law or for health authorities to give directives with which a majority of doctors disagree (or even a majority of the public disagree when a voting system can give a party a massive majority with less than 50 per cent of the popular vote). The power, limitations and role of the law will be discussed in the next chapter. There is at present considerable agreement within the profession but differences are appearing over the ethics of patient-assisted suicide, cloning and the use of stem cells. If doctors cannot agree, then there is pressure for regulation to be imposed from outside.

WHO MAKES THE RULES?

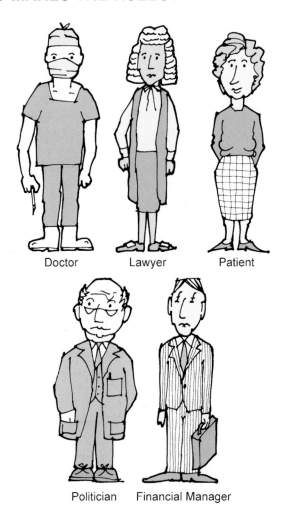

Doctor   Lawyer   Patient

Politician   Financial Manager

Should politicians, lawyers, managers, patients or doctors and their regulatory bodies make the rules? The answer is that all groups have some input, because politicians pass laws governing medical practice, lawyers administer them and take doctors to court, and patients are being increasingly represented on official and professional committees. In the UK the General Medical Council (GMC) is responsible for approving medical school curricula, for licensing doctors and monitoring their practice, and for disciplining them when they fall short of agreed standards. The key document is *Good Medical Practice* (GMC, 2001) and the GMC also publishes guidance on different problems such as *Withholding and Withdrawing Life-prolonging Treatment* (GMC, 2002a), *Research: The Role and Responsibility of Doctors* (GMC, 2002b) and *Confidentiality: Protecting and Providing Information* (GMC, 2004). The British Medical Association (BMA), the Medical Royal Colleges and the Medical Defence Associations also produce ethical guidance in their particular spheres and these often overlap.

OATHS, CODES AND DECLARATIONS

Over the years the profession has produced consensus statements on ethical matters. The most famous of these is the ancient Hippocratic Oath, which probably did not come from Hippocrates himself, but from a small group of Pythagorean doctors who wished to adopt standards higher than those around them. It certainly did not reflect the normal practice in ancient Greece. The Oath has a few simple ethical imperatives:

- To do no harm
- Not to assist suicide or administer euthanasia
- Not to cause abortion
- To refer patients to someone better qualified if necessary
- Not to abuse professional relationships, especially for sexual motives
- To keep patients' confidences.

Of course, the 1967 Abortion Act in the UK erased one of the main principles at a stroke.

The Oath also contains a duty to help out one's teachers financially and then to teach their children, if requested to do so. To modern ears these phrases sound like a blueprint for a nepotistic clique! Nevertheless, this document stood in splendid isolation for hundreds of years until the atrocities of Nazi Germany in the 1940s and the rapid growth of treatment possibilities in the twentieth century led to the modern spate of declarations and codes.

The Declaration of Geneva was the first of these, adopted by the General Assembly of World Medical Association (WMA) in 1948. It is an updated restatement of the Hippocratic Oath and was followed by the more detailed International Code of Medical Ethics in 1949. The WMA then produced a series of declarations on specific issues such as the Declaration of Helsinki on clinical research and human experimentation (updated 2003), which is more detailed than many of the others and serves as a standard for hospital research ethics committees. Other declarations include Sydney (1968) on the definition of death for transplantation, Oslo (1970) on therapeutic abortion, Tokyo (1975) on torture and Hawaii and Venice, etc. Each is named after the city in which the WMA was meeting and where the declaration was agreed.

For WMA declarations to become binding on an individual country, they have to be adopted by the national medical association, which in the UK is the BMA. It is a moot point whether international codes should have precedence over national directives. This may be important if a national government tries to insist on doctors behaving in what they consider an unethical way (e.g. being asked to take part in amputation of hands as punishment for theft, which contravenes the Declaration of Tokyo).

Although these declarations are not laws they carry considerable weight in law. For example if a patient dies during a clinical research project and the Helsinki guidance has not been followed, the coroner would not be impressed. Let us now look at some ethical conflicts that may arise in practice.

CONFLICTS

Conflict between doctor and doctor

Patients are increasingly treated by multidisciplinary teams of doctors and other health care workers and they may be referred from team to team. For example, a GP may recommend an abortion but the gynaecologist may disagree. In a country where euthanasia is legal, a family doctor may have promised to agree to the patient's wish to end her life but then she is referred to a surgeon and then, again, on to a palliative care team who take different views. She would like to stay under the palliative care team but wants her GP to be brought in when she requests physician-assisted suicide (PAS).

Whistle-blowing

What should a doctor do if he or she thinks a colleague is behaving unethically? Although the National Health Service (NHS) in the UK is supposed to have a transparent 'no blame' culture, it does not always feel like that if you speak out! The first step is to check the facts, because hospitals are renowned breeding grounds for rumours. Whistle-blowing for trivial unsubstantiated claims should be discouraged. There is an established chain of responsibility within hospitals but the decision to report rests on the stage at which the doctor's responsibility to the patient overrides the doctor's responsibility to good relationships with colleagues (which are also in the patient's best interest).

The most publicized recent case was in Bristol where an anaesthetist reported surgeons for their operative practice and results of major heart surgery in children. This led to huge publicity and a large public inquiry (Bristol Royal Infirmary Inquiry, 2001). In this case there was in fact no fundamental difference in the ethical aims between the doctors (i.e. to benefit the children and reduce harm). Neither side was saying, as some modern philosophers might, that children under 2 were not self-aware and so should not be regarded as fully human. The anaesthetist, however, thought the surgeons were not keeping to the ethical principles of not harming patients by their clinical decisions and operative techniques. By contrast, in another notorious case, some hospital doctors were investigated for not reporting Dr Shipman after one of his patients was admitted after he gave her a high dose of morphine. In addition, doctors are often slow to report colleagues who have clear alcohol problems which could endanger patients.

Conflicts between doctor and patient

The classic example of conflict between doctor and patient is a Jehovah's Witness's refusal on religious grounds to receive a life-saving blood transfusion. The doctor's ethical imperative is to do the patient good and not harm, but such patients put their spiritual salvation before their physical survival, believing that to receive somebody else's blood would risk eternal condemnation. The ethical and legal guidance is clear: the patient's autonomy is given precedence over the doctor's duty to save life, but it is a harrowing emotional experience for a doctor to see a patient die of haemorrhage knowing that he or she could have been saved by a blood transfusion. In the past, doctors found this so difficult that they sometimes put up a blood transfusion when patients were unconscious and replaced it with a saline drip before they woke up! Rather than being more ethical, this practice was just adding deception to the other ethical problems.

For children of Jehovah's Witnesses, the law overrules and the hospital usually applies to the County Court under the Children Act (1989) for a Specific Issue Order. Permission can be given rapidly by them contacting a High Court Judge by telephone who gives permission for a blood transfusion.

A recent example of conflict between doctor and patient concerned the parents of a severely handicapped child, Charlotte Wyatt, who insisted that doctors should put her on a ventilator if she developed respiratory failure, whereas the doctors thought that to do this repeatedly was inappropriate and futile treatment for a patient whose prognosis was so poor. The hospital ethics committee had been consulted but the parents went to court in a blaze of publicity and the court found in favour of the doctors. The parents then appealed to the High Court which overturned this ruling, partly because Charlotte's condition had improved unexpectedly. The Judge concluded 'that the treating doctor does not **take** orders from the family any more than he **gives** them. He acts in what he sees as the best interest of the child – no more, no less.'

Conflict between government, management and doctors

Parliament may pass laws governing health care with which many doctors may disagree. Conflict is now arising over guidelines, priority and targets from the managers of the Health Service. Governments are interested in political targets, whereas doctors are usually more concerned about the welfare of their own patients. For example, the present government has promised that no patient will wait more than one year for an operation (however trivial the condition). As the year-end approaches, patients with minor problems are given priority over patients with far more serious illnesses in order to keep a political promise. Many doctors find this unethical and difficult to implement (see Chapter 10 for further discussion).

Another serious problem for doctors is when a particular patient is used as a political pawn during an election campaign. On one occasion many years ago, the Prime Minister of the day, having been told about a baby with a heart problem, who had been waiting for surgery for some time, put pressure on the surgeons to expedite the operation. The baby died after the operation.

Another dilemma for doctors is to know when to refuse to admit patients or operate on them when the conditions in the hospital have deteriorated to levels which they consider dangerous. Does the surgeon 'make do' with poor alternatives when important equipment is not working? Should the physician go on admitting patients to a severely under-staffed ward? These dilemmas are, sadly, beginning to emerge in the UK NHS.

Managers have their own challenges because they are caught between political masters and accountants, angry doctors and needy patients. The answer to these conflicts is to have agreement on priorities and contingencies, before the crisis comes, but often these potential problems are not faced or discussed in a meaningful way.

CONSCIENCE CLAUSES

Traditionally, when faced with contentious moral issues doctors have been allowed to exercise the right not to agree to a treatment that is against their conscience. When the Abortion Act was implemented in 1967 it included a 'conscience clause' which stated that a doctor who had a conscientious objection should refer the patient to a colleague who did not. There is a similar clause in the 2004 draft of the Assisted Dying for the Terminally Ill Bill, but this was altered in the Bill that was blocked by the House of Lords in 2006 to 'If an attending physician ... has a conscientious objection ... the patient shall be free to consult another physician who does not'. There was also a clause saying there was no obligation on any hospital, hospice or nursing home to permit assisted death on its premises.

Julian Savulescu argues that 'a doctor's conscience has little place in the delivery of modern medical care' and 'should not be tolerated'. 'Doctors who compromise the delivery of medical services to patients on conscience grounds must be punished' (Savulescu, 2006). He suggests that people should not enter the profession unless they are prepared to undertake certain commitments.

There may be a case for disciplining a doctor who fails to give life-saving treatment but those Acts with conscience clauses hardly come into that category! One can sympathize with a Health Authority trying to provide a new 'service' if many doctors do not wish to take part; after the 1967 Act a number of gynaecologists opposed to abortion had difficulty in getting consultant jobs. The problem with Savulescu's argument is that doctors enter the profession on the basis of its ethics at the time and then find that Parliament changes the rules while they are in practice. In May 2006 at least two-thirds of physicians and general practitioners and over 90% of palliative care doctors were against a change in the law to permit assisted dying. So, if a law were passed, Savulescu's approach would lead to a majority of the profession being punished for non-compliance! Perhaps we should ask all prospective medical students, at interview, to promise to be prepared to end the lives of old people in nursing homes just in case, at some time in the future, a government rules that their lives are not worth living and it is too expensive to keep them alive. This idea will be music to the ears of totalitarian regimes world-wide and seriously undermines a doctor's autonomy and integrity.

In conclusion, there is still a wide measure of agreement on ethical matters within the profession, although this may be changing. However, different doctors may interpret the guidance differently in practice, which can lead to conflict. In a few situations there may be direct disagreement between patient and doctor, which is usually decided in the patient's favour if it does not commit the doctor to doing something against his or her own conscience. In the case of children, the courts are often involved. Political targets may increasingly conflict with doctors' duty of care, based on need.

Summary

- There is general agreement on most aspects of medical ethics at present.
- The Hippocratic Oath is the best known ancient guide to medical ethics
- The World Medical Association has agreed international Codes and Declarations.
- Politicians, lawyers, managers, patients and doctors all have an important input.

- In the UK the General Medical Council is responsible for licensing and monitoring doctors.
- Doctors may occasionally disagree with patients, managers or other doctors on ethical matters.
- They have a responsibility to resist or expose unethical practice.
- The courts may have to arbitrate in disagreements between doctors and patients.
- The courts may have to step in to protect children if parents refuse consent.
- Conscience clauses are an important safeguard of a doctor's integrity and autonomy.

6

LAW AND ETHICS

Law and ethics are distinguishable but interact in many ways. What is **legal** may still be **unethical** because law provides the outside limits to unethical behaviour, but is not good at ensuring and encouraging the finer points of ethics in everyday practice. The aim of this chapter is to demonstrate the interface between law and ethics illustrated by some important and relevant cases.

The two main divisions of law are criminal and civil. A doctor (or Hospital Trust) is usually taken to a civil court by a patient accusing them of negligence, but if the negligence or mistake is very serious the doctor could be tried for manslaughter in a criminal court. One of the important differences between the two is the burden of proof: in a criminal court the proof must be beyond reasonable doubt, whereas, in a civil court, it is the balance of probabilities, even if this is 51 per cent to 49 per cent. Of course, a doctor can be guilty of crimes even though they are committed in the surgery, as in the case of Harold Shipman. In English law there is a hierarchy of different courts, the higher being able to overrule the lower (see Figure 6.1).

Medical litigation always starts in the County Court. In order to obtain the judgement he or she wishes the patient may appeal to increasingly higher courts if given leave to do so. For example in 2001/2002, Diane Pretty, a woman in the late stages of motor neurone disease, wanted permission for her husband

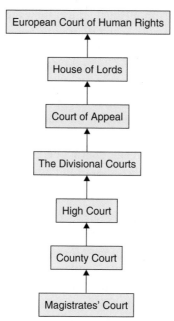

Figure 6.1 Hierarchy of civil courts in England and Wales (Note that the Scottish legal system differs in a number of ways.)

to help her end her life without being prosecuted for murder. She took her case right up to the European Court of Human Rights, which confirmed the judgement of the House of Lords that she did not have a right to be killed. She died of natural causes a short time later. The ethical issue here was autonomy (or patient's rights) and the European Court confirmed that autonomy was not absolute (see Chapter 7).

THE LAW'S INFLUENCE ON MEDICAL ETHICS

In the UK Parliament passes Acts on medical issues such as the Abortion Act (1967) or Mental Capacity Act (2005). This is known as statute law and normally carries a penalty or sanctions.

Parliamentary Bills on medical ethical topics may be introduced into the House of Lords or the House of Commons by private members (as with the Abortion Law) or more commonly by the Government of the day. Frequently this follows the deliberations of a Special Advisory Group or Committee, which makes recommendations. For example the Warnock Committee (1984) produced guidance which led to the Human Fertilisation and Embryology Act (1990), which gave clear guidance on *in vitro* fertilization, storage of eggs, sperm and embryos and research on embryos. Votes on these issues in Parliament are often left to a free vote rather than along party lines.

Second, the courts give judgements on individual cases to allow a treatment to be given or withheld. This is known as case or common law and a very good example is the judgement in 1993 of the House of Lords in the case of Anthony Bland, who was a young man in a persistent vegetative state following an injury at the Hillsborough football stadium disaster. The doctors were seeking permission to withdraw artificial nutrition and hydration.

The importance of case law is that judgements usually act as precedents for future similar cases and a higher court's judgement has priority over that of a lower court. Sometimes an individual judgement is made with the express statement that it should not be a precedent for future cases and that each should be treated on its merits at the time.

Indeed, one motive for a patient bringing a case to court is to create a precedent for the future. For example, in 2004 Leslie Burke, a patient with cerebellar ataxia, went to the High Court to challenge the guidance of the General Medical Council (GMC) that doctors could withdraw artificial nutrient and hydration when they could no longer prolong his life because he feared that they might do it before the final stages of his disease. The High Court declared that the section in the GMC guidelines about withdrawing artificial nutrient and hydration was unlawful, but in 2005 the GMC went to the Court of Appeal

and the judgement was overturned. In giving judgement, Lord
Phillips (the Master of the Roles) reassured him that there were
no grounds for him to think that those caring for him would
withdraw artificial nutrient and hydration in such circumstances – a position endorsed by the President of the GMC.

CORONERS' COURTS

The purpose of a Coroners' Court is to determine the mode and
cause of a patient's death and the doctor giving evidence is not
on trial. Nevertheless, if the doctor has made a significant mistake, the witness box can feel uncomfortably like the dock! The
Coroner does have the power to refer a doctor to a criminal court
if the findings suggest that a criminal act has taken place and a
doctor may be represented in the Coroners' Court by a lawyer.

In Scotland the Procurator Fiscal has a similar, but not identi-
cal, role to the Coroner in England and Wales.

THE GENERAL MEDICAL COUNCIL

The GMC is the appointed body to oversee training and to
license doctors to practice. Its committees are made up of lay
members as well as doctors. It is also responsible for monitoring standards and it has a disciplinary committee to examine
when doctors have fallen short of high ethical standards. It is
not part of the legal system but its guidelines are taken seriously by the courts. One of the problems is that the GMC is
both prosecutor and judge but a doctor does have legal
representation. Its most severe sanction is to strike a doctor
off the Medical Register – so ending his or her medical career.
Alternatively a doctor may be suspended for a year or more,
reprimanded or ordered to undergo further training.

The decision of the GMC may be overturned by a court. This
happened recently when the GMC suspended a highly skilled
plastic surgeon for 'unprofessional conduct' because he had

supposedly indulged in sexual relations with a patient. Partly due to pressure from his other patients and colleagues, an appeal was made to the High Court and the GMC suspension was over-ruled on the ground that many patients would be deprived of his exceptional skills. The GMC's published guidance can also be challenged in court, as in the case of Leslie Burke (see above).

Fitness to practice

Doctors, like anyone else, may become mentally ill or develop drug or alcohol dependence and may lose insight into their condition. The GMC has a Health Committee which looks into these matters and is separate from the Disciplinary Committee.

PRECEDENT

The precedent that has had the most far-reaching effect regard-ing a doctor's duty of care and negligence, is that of Bolam (1957). This case (in which the patient suffered a fractured hip while undergoing electroconvulsive therapy without adequate muscle relaxation) established that a doctor is not negligent if he or she acts in accordance with a responsible body of medical opinion, even if it is a minority opinion. This set a precedent, which is known as the 'Bolam test'. However, in 1997, in the case of Bolitho v. City and Hackney Health Authority, a Law Lord went further and ruled that such 'a responsible body of medical opinion had to demonstrate that their opinion was logical and reasonable and could withstand logical analysis'. Therefore the courts now have a role in evalu-ating the medical opinion, rather than accepting it uncritically.

The old adage 'Hard cases make bad laws' still holds true when individual cases produce precedent and authorities overreact to individual problems by producing multitudes of rules and regu-lations. There is no reason why a one-off exception to an ethical principle should lead to a generalized change in the law. For example, an often-quoted example in the euthanasia debate is

known as the 'policeman's dilemma': A motor accident leaves a
lorry driver trapped in his burning cab. He cannot be freed, so
signals to a policeman standing by to shoot him before he burns
to death. Many people would say the policeman is not wrong to
comply with his request; but to conclude from that one, exceptional situation that euthanasia should be legal for all terminally
ill patients, is an unjustified generalization, especially as their
pain is usually well controlled by skilled palliative care.

THE PROBLEM OF POLICING STATUTE LAW

It is relatively easy to pass a law through Parliament, but far
more difficult to police it and ensure it is not abused, especially as it is difficult to frame a law with enough detail to
anticipate every situation. There is genuine anxiety about 'slippery slopes' – that safeguards will be breached and indications
expanded. This concern was not helped by the 1967 Abortion
Act, which was in a sense an amendment to the old 1861
Offences Against the Person Act that made abortion a crime.
The 1967 Act states that abortion is not a crime under certain
conditions (but outside those conditions it still is). However the
wording of the Act was so imprecise that it rapidly led to virtu-
ally abortion on demand. One criterion – 'that the continuation
of the pregnancy would involve risk to the life of the pregnant
woman greater than if the pregnancy were terminated' – can
nearly always be fulfilled because early abortions in a fully
equipped hospital are now so safe.

The other problem in all Acts is the interpretation of individual
phrases, such as 'the child would suffer from such physical or
mental abnormalities as to be seriously handicapped'. What does
'serious' mean? An abortion for a relatively mild (remediable)
physical abnormality has recently been challenged in court.

On the other hand, the upper limit of 24 weeks is easier to
police and is not liable to the 'slippery slope' argument. Even

so there have been recent moves to lower this age limit because advances in neonatal intensive care have enabled babies delivered under 24 weeks to survive.

The 'slippery slope' argument has also been behind many of the objections to legalizing physician-assisted suicide. Even if it were defined carefully enough to be truly voluntary, there are still pitfalls. Lord Walton summed up the Select Committee's conclusions in 1994: 'We were also concerned that vulnerable people – the elderly, lonely, sick or distressed – would feel pressure, whether real or imagined, to request early death' (Walton, 1994).

The widening of the scope of statutes is sometimes produced by Amendments or new Acts in a stepwise progression, with each step being carefully defined. For example physician-assisted suicide could be applied initially to those with terminal illness and then be extended to those much earlier in the illness process and then perhaps by combining the Mental Capacity Act to those with mental incapacity, who have given advanced directives many years before they become ill.

On the other hand, the Human Fertilisation and Embryology Act (1990) was set up with the powers to regulate, monitor and inspect units undertaking *in vitro* fertilization and this has, on the whole, provided very effective policing.

THE PROBLEM OF LITIGATION

It is entirely appropriate that patients should have some recourse to compensation for medical mistakes. However, litigation has got completely out of hand in the USA and is becoming a major influence in the practice of medicine in the UK, where the National Health Service (NHS) now plans for over £6 billion each year to pay for possible damages. In some states in the USA, doctors are paying more in insurance premiums against damages than a British consultant's total salary. Recently, in the State of Mississippi, litigation was so bad that doctors were leaving the State at a rate that threatened the

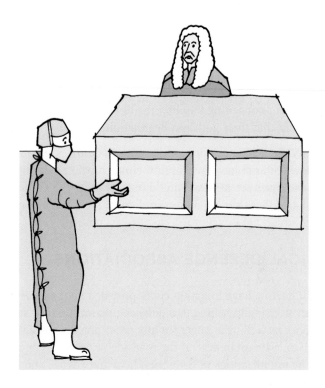

whole health care system. Only an intensive medical campaign persuaded the State Legislature to limit the power of lawyers.

Clearly, litigation leads to defensive medicine and overinvestigation and treatment that is not in the patient's best interest and therefore unethical. The fear of being sued may also prevent a surgeon from operating on a high-risk patient with a low but real chance of success. On the principle of fairness, the large amount of money paid out in damages may be unethical because it prevents or delays the treatment of many others. Then some patients who 'deserve' compensation may not receive it because they are unable to prove negligence.

In the UK many cases of litigation no longer come to court because of the Woolf Rules (1999) for Civil Procedure in County Courts and High Courts. These give time scales and ensure that the expert witnesses instructed by the two sides meet and try to agree their evidence. The other practical factor that stops cases coming to court is financial: a defending Hospital Trust simply decides whether it is cheaper to settle and give limited damages than to pay the legal fees of a court case. Although they may settle without conceding liability, the doctors concerned cannot help feeling that their guilt has been admitted.

To overcome these problems, at least two countries, Sweden and New Zealand, have a 'no fault' compensation system where the cases are assessed and damages (if any) awarded by a tribunal rather than an adversarial court system. This has distinct advantages except for lawyers' incomes!

MEDICAL DEFENCE ASSOCIATIONS

Hospital doctors have litigation cover provided by their hospital trust but still should belong to a defence organization for support and advice as well as to cover for any other practice outside the hospital or 'Samaritan acts' at the roadside or on-board an air-craft. The organizations provide legal help and advice, and they also offer ethical guidance on certain issues, and can often help to prevent litigation by advising timely explanations to patients.

THE LAW CAN OVERRIDE ETHICAL PRINCIPLES

The law can demand that a doctor breaks certain ethical obliga-tions to his or her patients for the sake of the public good. A good example is the requirement under the Public Health (Control of Diseases) Act 1984 to report certain infectious dis-eases to the local Public Health Authorities, even though this breaks the patient's confidence. A psychiatrist as a witness in court where a patient is being tried for a criminal offence may be asked to divulge highly confidential information obtained through the therapeutic relationship. If the doctor refuses, he or she may be held in contempt of court and can even be given a prison sentence. Similarly, doctors have to obey court orders to produce information or face the consequences. However, a doctor in an A&E department is not necessarily obliged to give a patient's clinical details to a policeman except to provide the name and address of a driver suspected of having committed an offence.

The Mental Capacity Act (2005) gives legal authority to a patient's advanced directives and confers enduring power of attorney to another person to make decisions on his or her behalf, should the patient lack mental capacity and be unable to make a decision. This might involve treatment which the doctors think would benefit the patient, but that the patient has previously indicated he or she would not want. It is an extension of the principle of autonomy and consent.

PUBLIC POLICY

Some public policy is in the form of statute but much policy affecting the NHS is in the form of guidelines and directives. These do not have the same force of law. If they seem unreasonable or unfair (inequitable) and are not in the best interest of some patients doctors have the right to refuse to comply, provided of course that this does not contravene the terms and conditions of their employment. As with statutes, hopefully there will have been consultation with the profession but doctors 'at the coalface' often feel they have little influence.

Summary
- Law and ethics are separable but closely related.
- A doctor's practice is not exempt from criminal law.
- Some ethical practices are enshrined in statute law.
- Many decisions are based on case law and precedent.
- Individual cases may be taken up a hierarchy of courts.
- The law can override ethical principles if it is in the public interest.
- Litigation is a very expensive and often unsatisfactory way of settling disputes.

7

AUTONOMY AND CONSENT

In the next five chapters we look in more detail at the five main ethical principles – in alphabetical order rather than in order of importance. The hierarchy and priorities will be discussed in Chapter 12.

AUTONOMY IN THEORY

Autonomy (from the Greek for 'self law' or 'rule') is the right of patients to make decisions about their treatment free from controlling interference from others, and from personal limitations that prevent a meaningful choice. It is summarized by the couplet 'I am the master of my fate, I am the captain of my soul'. The opposite is paternalism (from the Greek for 'father'), when a doctor decides what is best and carries it out with minimal consent. Some modern writers advocate absolute personal autonomy as the sole basis for medical ethics but John Gray considers the idea of 'free will' as a central mistake of Christianity, perpetuated by humanism and dismisses autonomy outright: 'the lesson of cognitive science is that there is no self to do the choosing' (Gray, 2002, page 115)!

The caricature of the arrogant, overbearing, non-listening hospital consultant may have been true in the past, but there has

been a huge swing towards patient autonomy over the last 50
years which may have gone too far. Paternalism is not necessarily bad – there are bad fathers but also good fathers who are
kind and caring and there are times when patients cannot
exercise autonomy because they are very ill and paternalism
has to step in.

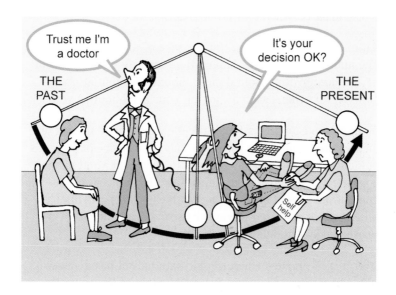

Are there limits to autonomy?

Absolute personal autonomy sounds fine, but other patients also
have rights. When does autonomy become selfishness? American
author LR Churchill has pointed out that extreme autonomy is
destroying the health system in the USA because fairness and
equity (see Chapter 10) are being denied (Churchill, 1987). Many
of those who champion 'absolute' autonomy qualify this by
adding 'as long as you do not harm or threaten anybody else's
person or property'. Others would agree that people's autonomy
should only be restricted to prevent harm to others, not harm to
themselves, because autonomy implies the freedom to make

wrong choices. In practice it is very difficult to make any decision that does not affect other people, either at the time or subsequently. For example, one patient demanding a very expensive and not very effective chemotherapy regime may stop another having a new and effective antibiotic in nine months' time when funds run out. Or the autonomy that demands physician-assisted suicide for one person may lead many years later to pressure on others to agree, when they do not really want to.

Autonomy can be 'limited' for the sake of the common good. The main religions (see Chapter 4) all identify with a concept of autonomy within boundaries – boundaries that also allow concern for others, such as 'loving your neighbour as yourself'.

Some health care professionals use the word 'client' instead of 'patient' in the mistaken belief that this emphasizes the patient's autonomy and reduces paternalism. However, the word patient comes from a Latin word meaning 'to suffer' whereas client comes from a word meaning 'a person who is dependent on others' patronage'. That is why we use the word patient unashamedly throughout this book!

One area of practice where classic paternalism has given way to a partnership of consent is Do Not Attempt Resuscitation (DNAR) orders. These used to be the prerogative of the health care team but are now openly discussed with patients before being signed.

AUTONOMY IN PRACTICE

Consent for treatment

To operate on a patient without his or her consent is 'assault and battery' and against the law. However the word consent is unfortunate, in that it implies a reluctant agreement to an action decided by someone else (i.e. acceding to a request).

Alistair Campbell, formerly Professor of Medical Ethics at
Bristol University, has pointed out that the boot is really on the
other foot – it is the patient who is asking for the treatment
and the doctor who is consenting; we should, he suggests, talk
about request for treatment (Johnson, 2001). He agrees that
consent is the right word for a patient involved in a research
project, which has, indeed, been devised by someone else.
Although there may be no legal differences, there is a difference in the attitudes that the words reflect. However, the word
consent is in current usage and is usually qualified by the word
'informed' or 'valid'.

Can consent be truly informed?

No-one can really be fully informed about the benefits and
risks of a procedure – indeed the doctor may not know the
risks for that particular patient. In the USA, a consent form
contains great detail of even very small risks. In the UK, the
law accepts that the doctor's duty is to inform the patient of
the main benefits and common or significant risks. The patient
then agrees to the operation on the understanding that the
nature and effects of the operation have been explained. For
patients to be truly informed, the explanation must be in terms
that mean something to them – not a mishmash of Greek and
Latin jargon! When explaining intestinal obstruction to a
plumber, we do not need to describe the physiology of the gastrointestinal tract: he knows perfectly well what a blocked pipe
means!

Nevertheless, the information must be relevant to the particular
patient. For example, an operation on the hand that could
leave an interphalangeal joint with restricted movement would
not represent an important or significant risk to a footballer
but would be of great significance to a concert pianist. Similarly,
the risk associated with a thyroid operation, with a 1–2 per cent
chance of damaging the nerve to the vocal cords, would not be

as important for a shepherd (who controls his dogs by whistling) as to a professional singer.

The doctor still has discretion to decide how much to tell, while leaving opportunity for the patient to ask more. It might be appropriate to omit details of small risks, for example, which might only serve to frighten the patient and lead to a refusal to have the operation.

A patient awaiting a standard varicose vein operation on a hospital ward was told by a pre-registration house officer that one of the risks of the operation is bleeding to death! She immediately packed her bags and left the hospital.

Although bleeding to death could occur, it is extremely unlikely – indeed she had more risk of bleeding to death from accidental damage to her untreated varicose veins. Hence consent for operation should be obtained by a surgeon senior enough to be able to explain and answer questions, ideally, by the operating surgeon in person.

It is important to note that the detail of consent in the UK is rapidly approaching that of the USA. The amount of detail given will also depend on the urgency and seriousness of the procedure. If a patient needs an emergency operation to control severe gastrointestinal bleeding, the length of the scar or whether the patient will be left with some indigestion afterwards is of no importance compared with the results of not having the operation (i.e. death). On the other hand, if a patient is undergoing a non-urgent, cosmetic operation, he or she must be given every detail of even minor side-effects and the likely appearance of the scars.

It is essential to note on the consent form, and in the patient's notes, the information that has been given: if a severe complication should occur, the patient or relatives cannot say they would not have agreed to the operation if they had known the risks.

> No one can give consent on behalf of another adult unless he or she has enduring power of attorney.

The famous legal case that tested the amount of information that should be given to patients was that of Sidaway (1984). This involved a woman who underwent an operation for a slipped disc but was left with a damaged spinal cord, causing some paralysis of her arm. She sued the hospital on the grounds that she had not been told of this risk, even though it was small. The case went from the High Court to the Court of Appeal and finally to the House of Lords (see Chapter 6) which rejected it by a majority decision on the basis of the Bolam test.

More recently, courts have also been applying the Bolitho test (page 72) under which the information included is what a reasonable patient might wish to know, rather than what a doctor might decide to tell.

> *There is an alternative paradigm ... the expert–expert relationship ... the professional is the expert on treatment options ... but the patient is an equally valid expert, with specialist knowledge in his or her personal concerns.*
>
> (Wyatt, 1998, page 233)

Autonomy includes the right not to know

Can a patient transfer his or her autonomy to the doctor? Many older patients do not want to make choices about their treatments and say 'You are the doctor, do not confuse me with lots of details – just fix it' (the sort of attitude that some of us have to a reliable car mechanic!). Or they ask 'Which treatment would you have, doctor, if you were me?' After all, they have come for advice to an expert they trust. This is perfectly ethical but puts the onus on the doctor and there is a danger that in our desire to promote autonomy we put the burden of decision onto the patient which should be borne by the professional.

To take an illustration from another walk of life, when flying to New York do you want the pilot to tell you all the technical problems that might arise on the trip and the times he has had difficulty landing at JFK Airport? You do not sign a consent form every time you get on an plane; you just buy a ticket and walk onto the plane voluntarily, trusting in the skills of the crew and the efficiency of the machinery and knowing that the mortality rate is very low. Like a patient undergoing an anaesthetic a passenger cannot suddenly decide half way across the Atlantic that he or she no longer wants to continue the journey!

Autonomy means the right to refuse

Adult patients have the perfect right to refuse treatment even though doing so might endanger their life and health. The doctor's responsibility is to ensure that he or she has explained the dangers of refusing in a way that the patient can understand. If the doctor doubts that the patient has the capacity either to understand or make a decision, a psychiatric or second opinion must be obtained urgently. If the doctor thinks that the patient is just frightened or confused, he or she can offer to return later and discuss it further, and always allow for a change of mind. However much a doctor is committed to patient autonomy, it is still difficult to watch a patient that could have been cured leave the ward without treatment.

Implied consent

There are many minor procedures, including physical examination, for which no formal consent is obtained. If a patient voluntarily visits the doctor and holds out a hand to show a ganglion, for example, it is assumed that the patient has given implied consent for an examination. Similarly, if a doctor says a blood test is needed, giving the reasons, and the patient puts out an arm and allows the doctor to put on a tourniquet, it can be justly assumed that the patient is giving consent for the blood to be taken. However, it is wise to ask for specific verbal consent before intimate examinations such as those of the rectum or vagina (see also Chapter 15).

A Muslim woman came to a clinic complaining of a breast lump and was seen by a male surgeon who asked if he could examine her breast, but she refused. There was no female consultant in the hospital, so the surgeon asked a female junior doctor to examine and report her findings. He decided to operate on the basis of these, but in the theatre found that the lump was different and larger than he expected and needed a larger operation. What should he have done before and during the operation?

Capacity or competence to consent

Some patients obviously do not have the capacity to consent because they are unconscious and under these circumstances the doctors have to take the decision which they believe is in the patient's best interest. Relations can advise and express opinions, but cannot give consent. Some patients may be going in and out of consciousness and others may just be confused, but may still be able to understand enough to give consent.

> Just because someone is legally detained under a Section of the Mental Health Act, it does not imply that he or she is incapable of giving consent for an operation.

The Mental Capacity Bill (2005) clarifies the situation by allowing advanced directives and arranging enduring power of attorney, before a patient lacks capacity. In Scotland it is a little different (Adults with Incapacity Act 2000).

Consent for children

In England and Wales, young people under 18 but over 16 years of age can give consent to treatment, but cannot harm themselves severely by refusing treatment (Family Law Reform Act, 1969). Children under 16 can also give consent if they can understand the facts. This is referred to as 'Gillick competence' after a case in 1985 in which Victoria Gillick, challenging the Health Authority's advice to doctors to prescribe contraception for children under 16 without their parents' knowledge, was defeated by a House of Lords judgement. (In Scotland, a child under the age of 16 can give consent if a doctor is satisfied that the child can understand the nature and effects of the operation.) For example, if an 11-year-old child whose parents want him or her to have cosmetic surgery for bat ears does not want such surgery, the doctor can accept the child's refusal. On the other hand, if the child refuses a life-saving procedure or one that would prevent severe harm, the parents can override the child's refusal.

A particularly difficult example is that of profoundly deaf parents refusing permission for a cochlear implant for their baby to enable the child to hear, saying that deafness is not a disease to be corrected. Unfortunately, to be successful, the operation has to be done when the child is very young and one wonders what children's reactions will be when they grow up and become 'competent'.

Pressure to consent

Patients can be put under considerable pressure by relatives, friends and sometimes the health care team to agree to an operation or treatments that they really do not want to have. An example of this is when someone in renal failure needs a kidney transplant and either a relative is 'suggested' by the family to donate the kidney or, as happens in some countries, members of the public are paid to donate or prisoners bribed by the promise of early release. The tea and biscuits given to blood donors can hardly be considered coercive! A doctor's duty is to ensure that as far as possible consent is truly voluntary (payment for research studies will be discussed in Chapter 12).

> For consent to be valid, the patient must be informed, competent and take the decision voluntarily.

Consent for clinical research

In a clinical research context the disclosure of facts may be more detailed than in a treatment context, and here the word 'consent' is more appropriate. When a procedure or investigation has no direct benefit to the patient or may even be potentially harmful, every detail of the risk must be given. The Declaration of Helsinki (2003) provides guidance on clinical research with patients and normal volunteers. Research protocols are designed to ensure maximum benefit and reduce any harm and, in recent years, patients have been increasingly involved in the planning and design of research studies. The concept of doctors researching on patients has been replaced by the idea of patients and doctors being partners in the research enterprise, which is a far healthier balance of paternalism and autonomy. The Medical Research Council has given important guidance on the ethics of clinical research (MRC, 2005).

Use of placebos

If one of the ethical principles is to do good, is it ethical to use a dummy medicine (placebo) or even a placebo operation? It is only ethical to use a placebo if (a) there is a fair chance of a placebo response (i.e. symptoms improving) and (b) there is a fair chance of side-effects from the active drug which those in the placebo group will avoid. If there is standard treatment for a condition, a new treatment is usually compared with that – but ideally it should be a double-blind, randomized trial to exclude the placebo response of the new and perhaps hyped-up treatment. However, the important ethical principle with placebos is that the patients are aware that they are being used and that they have a 50:50 chance of receiving it. An example is discussed in Chapter 14.

Research on tissues removed at operation and post mortem

For many years it was accepted that a diseased organ removed from a patient could be used for ethical research (but not sold or used to establish cell lines) without special permission because the patient was deemed to have discarded it. To remove any other tissues the surgeon had to obtain specific permission. The Alder Hey Inquiry (Royal Liverpool Children's Inquiry, 2001) into the retention of babies' organs after post mortem for later research (into cot death) led to huge media coverage and probably an over-reaction by the authorities. It subsequently led to the Human Tissue Act (2004) and the setting up of the Human Tissue Authority to oversee it. Full implementation was in April 2006 and it details the particular consent needed in each situation.

Research with children

Matters of consent and autonomy make clinical research with children very difficult. Indeed, the recent Alder Hay experience has meant that fewer families are taking part in research projects.

CONCLUSION

Does the growing emphasis on autonomy and consent imply a lack of trust in doctors? A good doctor–patient relationship with mutual respect and common goals for care are far more helpful than forms, regulations and litigation, but documentation is here to stay and procedures must be carefully followed.

Summary

- In the last 50 years there has been a huge swing from paternalism to patient autonomy.
- Autonomy without limitations becomes licence and selfishness.
- An effective health care system demands respect for each other's autonomy.
- Autonomy involves the right to refuse life-saving treatment.
- Valid consent must be informed, competent and without coercion.
- Children between the ages of 16 and 18 can give consent for treatment but cannot refuse it if there is a risk of serious harm.
- Special care is needed with consent for clinical research.

8

BENEFICENCE

Beneficence is an action and benevolence an attitude, of good towards another person. It seems almost an insult to have a whole chapter on, doing good, in a book for medical students and doctors. Surely no one would be in the medical profession if they did not at least want to do good for patients, even though they may also have many additional motives, such as making money and having a high status in society. The corollary of doing good is avoiding or preventing harm (non-maleficence). In some ways, doing harm or failing to prevent it is more serious and culpable than failing to maximize benefit. The Hippocratic obligation 'to do no harm' can also be understood as a 'fall-back position' when the treatments of the time could do very little good, and could be rephrased as 'if you can't do any good at least don't do any harm'. Nowadays the situation is very different in that many of our treatments are so powerful that they nearly all have potential for harm. There is no longer a duty just to do whatever we can; rather, we need to ask whether we **should** do what we can do, when there is a real chance of making the patient worse. Any treatment decision is a balance between the potential for good and the potential for harm and this is particularly relevant to major surgery or chemotherapy in the elderly in which there is a significant mortality rate.

On the other hand, modern medicine has been put on such an unrealistic pedestal that patients have come to think that it can and should, cure all illnesses. In fact, most treatments, whether medical or surgical, merely control one part of the disease or delay its progression. Coronary artery bypass, for example, deals with atheromatous narrowing of one or more of the coronary vessels but atheromatous disease is usually widespread and can later lead to ischaemia of the legs or brain. Interestingly, the upper limit of human life has not changed for thousands of years but modern medicine has enabled far more people to approach that upper limit. In the fifteenth century there was a simple motto for the aims of treatment: 'To cure sometimes, to relieve often, to comfort always'. Although we may think we have outgrown such a simplistic idea of beneficence, the principles are as true now as when they were written, even though we might change the motto to: 'To cure quite often, to relieve very frequently, to comfort always'.

One of the difficulties about 'doing good', especially when treating cancer, is to decide when to change from attempting to cure, often with painful and distressing side-effects, to palliation and concentrating on relieving symptoms. The obligations of beneficence and non-maleficence may be summarized in the following hierarchy.

- Do positive good
- Make sure good outweighs harm
- Prevent harm
- Do not directly harm.

What is good for the patient?

This is an important question about doing good that must be faced; how do we decide what is good for a patient? As we have pointed out already, medical science cannot answer that question. Eric Cornell, who won the Nobel Prize for physics in 2001, has put it like this:

> *Should scientists, as humans, make judgements on ethics, morals, values and religion? Absolutely.*

> *Should we act on these judgements, in an effort to do good? You bet. Should we make use of the goodwill we may have accumulated through our scientific achievements to help us do good? Why not? Just don't claim that your* science *tells you 'what is good' or 'what is God'.*
>
> (Cornell, 2005)

How then do we define what is good for patients? A good starting point is to say that anything that promotes health is good; but what is health?

GOOD HEALTH: THE GOAL OF MEDICAL CARE

In 1948, the World Health Organization (WHO) defined health as 'a state of complete physical, mental and social well-being and not merely absence of disease'. The importance of this definition is that it includes more than one aspect of what it means to be human. Health cannot be defined in terms of one anatomical attribute or physiological function. A patient may have perfectly normal routine blood tests but be in severe depression and socially deprived. The quote 'He died but his electrolytes were normal', attributed to a professor of metabolic medicine, is probably apocryphal but epitomizes a narrow view of health that has been prevalent in the past.

So beneficence must include the idea of promoting a patient's health in the broadest sense because, sometimes, physical health and mental well-being may be in competition. An heroic operation might improve physical health significantly, for example, but leave the patient with a severe reactive depression. Towards the end of the twentieth century, the WHO had the wildly optimistic slogan 'Health for all by the year 2000'. 'Access to health care' would have been more realistic.

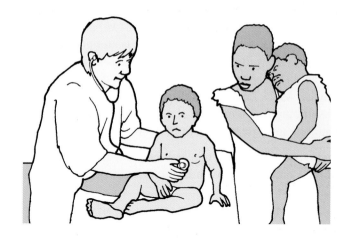

Social well-being

Interpersonal relationships are fundamental to being human, but social well-being is difficult to define. We may question a treatment of a physical disease that cuts a patient off from family and friends for long periods, it must be questioned. By the same token, lonely people, however physically fit, with no one who cares about them, cannot be said to be fully healthy; but if social well-being is defined in terms of lifestyle and possessions, how can anyone decide when it is complete? Is it the acquisition of a five-bedroomed house and two cars? What about the size of the TV set? Of course these things all depend on someone's expectations being satisfied.

Well-being and value systems

The different value systems referred to in Chapter 4 have different perspectives on what is meant by health and well-being. A utilitarian describes health and well-being in terms of pleasure (the hedonistic calculus) and so good health will be what enables the person to enjoy these pleasures. Others would point to the great creativity in art and music that has come as a result of suffering ill-health. Was Beethoven 'healthy' when he was profoundly deaf and mentally unstable, yet writing his Choral Symphony? Those with a religious value system would point to the increased spiritual awareness and deeper relationship with God acquired as a result of illness. That is not to claim that ill-health is good in itself but that it can produce good outcomes. As CS Lewis put it, 'God whispers in our pleasures, speaks in our conscience, but shouts in our pain: it is his megaphone to rouse a deaf world' (Lewis, 1940/2002, page 91).

A guide to potential different replies to the question 'What is good for a patient?' is given in Box 8.1.

Box 8.1 Various potential answers to the question 'What is good for a patient?'

- The follower of one of the main **monotheistic religions** says that good is what agrees with God's character of love and justice, and His will for that person.
- The **utilitarian** says that good is what gives the most pleasure.
- The **social Darwinist** says that good is what improves the quality of the human species.
- The **existentialist** says that good is what you feel is good at the time.
- The **individualist** says that good is what the patient wants.

'In the patient's best interest' – Who decides?

A doctor is obliged to act in the patient's best interest. When patients are fully competent, who judges what is in their best interests and on what criteria? The doctor may have a set of criteria that can be tested, such as physical mobility and cognitive assessment scores. Patients may be much more interested in how they feel about themselves (mental state) rather than any particular physical function. They may be much happier confined to a wheelchair than struggling to walk with the help of a Zimmer frame, even though their 'mobility scores' will be lower. In a previous generation one of the motives behind lying to patients about a bad diagnosis was to 'make them happy' because 'ignorance was bliss'. However, that is a very short-term view; when patients fail to get better and learn that they have been deceived, they may be anything but happy. Ill-health can be used both consciously and unconsciously to keep the attention of family and friends. Some patients even fake physical illness in order to increase their mental and social well-being.

On the other hand an Olympic athlete may be very healthy physically but his mental state and social relationships away from the stadium may be very 'unhealthy'.

There are times when a patient's view of best interest differs from that of the doctor. Patients may refuse a treatment which a doctor firmly believes is in their best interests and they have the right to do so (Chapter 7) or they may want the treatment despite the doctor's belief that it will not benefit them. In this case the doctor has the right to refuse. This may be a particular problem with requests for cosmetic surgery, or giving certain courses of chemotherapy which only prolong life for a few weeks at a significant cost in morbidity such as nausea, vomiting and hair loss.

Maximizing the patient's potential

Another approach to doing good is to help patients reach their physical, social and mental potential, even though these may be limited. A sense of well-being is related closely to ambition and expectation. A patient desperate to do a 10-mile sponsored walk will be frustrated and mentally unhealthy if claudication makes only a mile or two possible despite maximum treatment. If, on the other hand, the patient's ambition is limited to walking a quarter of a mile to the pub to have a drink with friends, even a slight improvement would give a sense of physical, mental and social well-being. It has been rightly pointed out that a huge amount of unhappiness and discontentment in modern Western society is due to people's expectations being continually increased by the media.

In the doctor's best interest?

One aspect of this whole question of beneficence is not in doubt: doctors must not act in their own best interests to the detriment of patients. For example, a surgeon may see a patient in his private clinic, who has had haemorrhoids for some time for which there is a choice of two possible treatments: simple banding in the clinic or an operation. The operation obviously brings a higher fee and the surgeon has to be detached from self-interest in order to give advice that is in the patient's best interest. Similarly in any private health system there is a strong incentive to do operations such as hysterectomy and appendicectomy for relatively slight symptoms. In the USA hospitals have tissue committees that check on the pathology of the organs removed to ensure that normal organs are not being removed unnecessarily. In a socialized health system such as the UK's National Health Service with long waiting lists for operations the incentive may be the opposite – to advise conservative treatment when an operation would in fact be in the patient's best interest.

Medical enhancement – super-humans

Until quite recently the efforts of medicine were directed to returning people to as normal a state as possible. This involved correcting anatomical defects, restoring abnormal physiology, eliminating disease and healing wounds and fractures. Rapid scientific advances are bringing close possibilities that have only previously been the domain of science fiction. Genetic enhancement and human/machine mergers (cyborgs) can in theory produce 'super-humans'. This approach is known as transhumanism and the movement is influential. It is based on the philosophy of rational humanism, which states that humans are still in the process of evolving and improving and that we can take control of our own destiny by applying new scientific knowledge.

Those with a religious value system take issue with this concept, because they believe humans to be a distinct, complete and special species, the crown of creation (by whatever process) with special accountability to God. Of course we all use scientific instruments such as microscopes or telescopes to enhance our normal eyesight, but transhumanists propose silicone chips implanted into a normally functioning brain that can carry thought processes without speech.

Ageing

The transhumanist Nick Bostrom considers the search for a cure for ageing to be an 'urgent, screaming, moral imperative' (Bostrom, 2005). Again we must ask whether there is a normal ageing process which is part of being human, albeit with abnormalities such as hip fractures and cataracts on the way, or whether ageing is part of the incompleteness of human development that should be corrected and prevented. This in turn begs the fundamental question: Is this life all that there is or is ageing and death a journey towards a more glorious changed life in the future? Or, put another way, are humans merely physical beings or do they have a spiritual and eternal component?'.

The key question is whether there is a significant ethical difference, for example, between using electronic equipment to enable a paraplegic patient to write using facial movements, and using electronic machines to enhance intelligence? Certainly the athletic world disapproves strongly of performance-enhancing drugs and the doctors who may prescribe them.

Ethical debate is based on first, the nature of being human (see Chapter 4) and, secondly, on equity and justice. This raises the practical question of whether it is right to spend huge sums on a few people being super-human when millions are in need of simple treatments to return them to normal.

TWO SCENARIOS

We will illustrate these issues with two quite different examples:

1. *A woman of 30 wishes to store her ova so that she can pursue a promising career and then have children by IVF in her mid-forties. She had heard that fertility rapidly declines around the age of 40 and she does not have a partner at present. This has been dubbed 'putting motherhood on ice'.*

When faced with this request, how does the doctor decide whether complying with the patient's request is in her best interest and for her good? First, we can say there is nothing intrinsically wrong with the principle. Many people would find storing ova far more acceptable than storing embryos. The large financial cost is a factor, but this particular patient would be prepared to pay. The problem of 'best interest' is in the difficulty of foreseeing the consequences. If the freezing and thawing is unsuccessful, for example, she will have missed her opportunity to conceive altogether. Other considerations are the family and social impact of older parents and, after another generation has followed suit, perhaps, no grandparents for a newborn child.

2. *An NHS Trust is £5 million overspent and has announced that hundreds of staff are to be made redundant. This could severely affect patient services and further diminish staff morale. Should doctors protest by going on strike?*

In several parts of the world in recent years doctors and other health workers have withdrawn their services – at least for elective work – to protest about pay and conditions or decisions taken by politicians. At first sight this is a direct conflict between what is in the best interest of the patient and what is to the advantage of the doctor. But doctors might argue that, in the long run, their action is in the best interest of the patient. If the pay and conditions are not improved, people will not come into medicine and there will be a severe shortage to treat future patients. They might also point out that a disgruntled care team does not function well and will not do the best for its patients. The problem of health care, as opposed to car manufacturing, is that it is impossible to hurt an employer without harming patients in some way. If, in exceptional circumstances, the profession considered it right to withdraw its services, it could only be ethical if arrangements were made to treat emergencies and the very ill, thus producing inconvenience rather than real danger to patients. But when the ambulance service goes on strike acutely ill patients are affected and the government has no alternative but to bring in army ambulances.

Another time that 'strike' action could be justified is if doctors were given instructions by politicians that they genuinely believed were not in the patients' best interests.

CONCLUSION

The concept of improving health and 'doing good' to people is as complex as human beings themselves. A simplistic answer is not satisfactory. Many aspects need to be considered and under-standing a patient's background, values, expectations and needs is essential. Varying components of beneficence are well summa-rized in the General Medical Council advice on deciding the best interest of a patient who lacks capacity (Box 8.2). It is important to note that **not** treating can be in the patient's best interest.

Box 8.2 'Best interests' principle

In deciding what options may be reasonably considered as being in the best interests of a patient who lacks capacity to decide, you should take into account:

● Options for treatment or investigation which are clinically indicated
● Any evidence of the patient's previously expressed prefer-ences, including an advance statement
● Your own and the health care team's knowledge of the patient's background, such as cultural, religious, or employ-ment considerations
● Views about the patient's preferences given by a third party who may have other knowledge of the patient, for example the patient's partner, family, carer, tutor-dative (Scotland), or a person with parental responsibility
● Which option least restricts the patient's future choices, where more than one option (including non-treatment) seems reasonable in the patient's best interest.

From GMC (1998).

Summary

- 'Doing good' and preventing harm are fundamental duties of a doctor.
- Medical science alone cannot determine what is good for a patient.
- Good health includes physical, mental, social and spiritual factors.
- Well-being can be defined by objective measurements, by patients' feelings or fulfilling expectations.
- It is debatable how much enhancing normal health is ethical.
- A patient may refuse treatment that a doctor considers to be in the patient's best interest.
- A doctor is not obliged to accede to a request for treatment which he or she does not think is in the patient's best interest.
- When a patient lacks capacity, the medical team must assess best interest by a series of clearly defined guidelines.

9

CONFIDENTIALITY

Confidentiality is perhaps the most familiar of all the doctors' ethical duties. It is a key part of the ancient Hippocratic Oath: 'Whatever in connection with my professional practice, or not in connection with it, I see or hear in the life of men which ought not to be spoken of abroad, I will not divulge as reckoning that all such be kept secret', as well as the Declaration of Geneva (1948/1994): 'I will respect the secrets which have been confided in me even after the patient has died'. Why is it so important?

The basis of any doctor–patient relationship is trust. A patient will only reveal sensitive, personal details that are essential for diagnosis and treatment, if confident that they will not be passed on to others. Doctors have been prepared to go to prison for contempt of court to protect a patient's confidentiality, but it is breached many times a day in every hospital by carelessness or by people trying to be too helpful.

COMMON BREACHES OF CONFIDENTIALITY

On open hospital wards, it is almost impossible to preserve confidentiality while talking to a patient. For sensitive discussions, doctors should find a private room, even if this means moving the patient in his or her bed.

It is easy to forget that curtains around a bed are not sound-proof.

Medical students and junior doctors love to discuss clinical details of patients they have seen on a ward round or in a clinic, and that is a learning process. But when this is done in the hospital lift or on the bus going home, confidentiality is easily breached. Another person within earshot could be a neighbour or a friend of the patient.

It is tempting for a student to text a friend when a particularly rare or interesting case has just been seen. Hospital notes are often left around on ward nursing stations or in waiting areas. Hospital porters may casually look through the notes while waiting for a lift and medical secretaries are in a particularly privileged position when typing letters and clinical details. How many confidential telephone calls from ward nursing stations or from GPs' receptionists are overheard? When apparently well-meaning relatives telephone to ask how a patient is doing, it is easy for a doctor or nurse to give unnecessary confidential details while trying to reassure.

A 40-year-old man was admitted to hospital with a minor head injury but under the influence of alcohol. His brother telephoned the following day to ask how he was and the nurse replied that the injury was not severe and he was now sober. When the patient returned home he found he had lost his job – his brother was also his employer.

When a celebrity is ill there is always tremendous pressure to divulge details. Journalists have been known to go to great lengths to get information, posing as relatives, clergy and even doctors. If a patient is unconscious and cannot agree to a statement, any doctor approached by the media should immediately contact the hospital public relations officer. Statements usually have to be limited to vague generalizations such as 'critical but stable' or 'improving and out of danger'.

> Hospital lifts are not the right place to discuss patients: their privacy must be respected.

Common ways in which confidentiality is breached are listed in Box 9.1.

Box 9.1 Common ways in which confidentiality is breached

- Talking to patients in an open ward
- Talking in lifts or corridors
- Text messages
- Hospital notes
- Telephone calls
- Receptionists in GP surgeries.

TELLING RELATIVES

We have singled out this topic because there is still serious misunderstanding amongst many members of the health care team. It is a breach of confidentiality to give the details of any conscious adult patient to relatives, however close and concerned, without the permission of the patient. In the past it was common practice, especially with the elderly, to tell the relatives first about a serious diagnosis, and then ask if they thought the patient might like to know! You can never assume that the relatives' motives are always right and, in many families, there are relationship problems: a patient may be close to one child but be estranged from another. It is not difficult to ask patients if they would like you to talk to their family and if so to whom. Sometimes they will ask you not to bother one family member with details of the illness but to tell another instead, which is fine.

If a patient is unconscious, then, as always, the doctor considers the best interest of the patient and may tell one or more of the relatives (usually the one stated on the notes as 'next of kin'). In Chapter 7 we discussed the misconception that relatives can give consent on behalf of another competent adult.

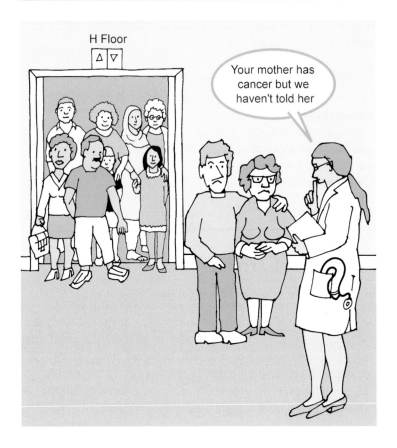

SAFEGUARDS

The key safeguard for confidentiality is to obtain the patient's permission, usually in writing, before divulging any information to a third party. A simple example is when a doctor is asked to fill in a form for a travel insurance company because a patient has been admitted to hospital and cannot go away on holiday. Even then the doctor should get written permission and only give information that is strictly necessary for that particular claim. Similarly, how much detail should a GP put on a 'sick note' which will go to a patient's employers? Finally, if you want to discuss your day's work with your spouse or friends, make sure you do not mention any patients' names, especially if they might know them.

Hospital records

Paper notes should be stored securely and only be available for staff authorized to see them. Computerized records and the results of tests are safeguarded by computer codes and differential access for different members of the care team. However, that does not mean that a house officer should obtain the results of a biopsy on a medical colleague who is on a different ward and under another doctor's care. You only have to be a patient in the hospital where you work to know how quickly confidentiality is breached!

Photographs, presentations and publications

Clinical photographs, particularly in publications, are a sensitive issue. Even if a patient cannot be identified because the photograph is of a lesion on a leg, it is still important to obtain written permission. When presenting or publishing case reports, only minimal information needs to be given and written patient permission should be requested before publication. Once details are published it is impossible to limit the spread of information, especially when it is available on the Internet. There is no need to give a patient's initials, such as 'Mrs H.B.'; 'a 40-year-old married woman', for example, is all that is needed.

Legal safeguards

It was not so long ago that patients' hospital notes had a notice on them 'Not be handled by the patient', such was the enthusiasm for concealing patients' health details from them! It was not until 1990 that the Access to Health Records Act gave patients the right to see what was in their notes and, even then, with some limitations at the doctor's discretion. This access has certainly stopped the previous, not uncommon practice of recording critical casual comments such as 'grumpy old man of 70'. However, it was the introduction of computers and the storage of vast amounts of information about people that led to the Data Protection Act in 1998. This Act sets out eight principles (Box 9.2).

Box 9.2   Data Protection Act – personal data

1. Personal data shall be processed fairly and lawfully, and, in particular, shall not be processed unless: (a) at least one of the conditions in Schedule 2 is met, and (b) in the case of sensitive personal data, at least one of the conditions in Schedule 3 is also met.
2. Personal data shall be obtained only for one or more specified and lawful purposes, and shall not be further processed in any manner incompatible with that purpose or those purposes.
3. Personal data shall be adequate, relevant and not excessive in relation to the purpose or purposes for which they are processed.
4. Personal data shall be accurate and, where necessary, kept up to date.
5. Personal data processed for any purpose or purposes shall not be kept for longer than is necessary for that purpose or those purposes.
6. Personal data shall be processed in accordance with the rights of data subjects under this Act.
7. Appropriate technical and organisational measures shall be taken against unauthorised or unlawful processing of personal data and against accidental loss or destruction of, or damage to, personal data.
8. Personal data shall not be transferred to a country or territory outside the European Economic Area unless that country or territory ensures an adequate level of protection for the rights and freedoms of data subjects in relation to the processing of personal data.

From Data Protection Act 1998.

Principle 8 is particularly relevant now that the typing of hospital letters is being outsourced to countries such as India. Principle 5 is also vital: for many years the National Confidential Enquiry into Patient Outcome and Death (formerly the National

Confidential Enquiry into Peri-Operative Deaths (NCEPOD) has collected details of patients who have died during or after different types of operations from all over the country. Patients' details are sent but they are anonymized as soon as they are received at the central office and then wiped off the computer once the analysis into the causes is complete. This fits well with the Declaration of Geneva's emphasis that the principle of confidentiality continues even after death.

EXCEPTIONS TO CONFIDENTIALITY

It is right and important to share information between doctors and other members of the health team and with GPs caring for the patient; this is done on the understanding that confidentiality will be preserved. Nevertheless, just because you are a doctor, it does not give you the right to information about a patient you are not treating, especially if you want to use it for publicity or political purposes. Sharing of confidences, even between doctors, must always be in the patient's interest.

Legal exceptions

There are certain situations in which doctors must breach confidentiality. These are summarized in Box 9.3.

Box 9.3   Compulsory breaches of confidentiality

- Births
- Deaths
- Notifiable disease
- Termination of pregnancy
- When there is a risk of harm to children
- To the police, if a patient is suspected of a road traffic offence (name and address only – not clinical details)
- Under court orders (including Coroners' Court)
- If there is a search warrant signed by a Circuit Judge.

The A&E department is a place where pressure is commonly put on doctors to break confidentiality when they should not.

For example, an enquiry by the police when there is no suspicion of a road traffic offence or a serious crime should be resisted.

An off-duty policeman was sitting in the outpatient department waiting room as a patient. He overheard two other patients discussing a burglary they had done! When one of the patients went forward to see the doctor the policeman identified himself to the receptionist and asked for the name of the patient. The receptionist, quite rightly, refused. If she had called out his name when his turn came, would she have been in breach of confidentiality?

Possible exceptions to confidentiality

Doctors are also citizens responsible to the wider population as well as their patients. When a serious crime, such as terrorism or murder, has been committed, doctors' responsibilities as citizens outweigh their duty of confidentiality to a patient. Similarly, if a patient with epilepsy continues to drive against advice, the doctor might need to tell the licensing authority. Persuasion should be tried first, rather than telling behind the patient's back, but if that fails the doctor has a duty to inform and should tell the patient accordingly. Psychiatrists are sometimes in a difficult situation if a patient admits an intention to commit a serious crime. They have to assess how likely this is, but may have to act for the safety of others. Sometimes it is wise not to promise absolute confidentiality to the patient (e.g. when discussing possible child abuse).

CONSEQUENCES OF HONOURING CONFIDENTIALITY

The policy of making records anonymous in the sexually transmitted diseases department can make it difficult to trace contacts or stop the spread of disease. Patients may be encouraged to advise their partners and contacts to seek treatment but if they refuse, should the doctor step in and warn a patient's spouse?

Under certain circumstances this can be justified for an individual case where risk is clear because the principle of preventing harm (see Chapter 8) overrides the duty to confidentiality.

The Data Protection Act, if applied rigorously, can make it impossible to keep details about patients for long enough to study epidemiology and long-term follow-up.

UNRESOLVED ISSUES

Family history

There has been a recent suggestion (Schmitz and Wiesing, 2006) that taking a family history could breach the relatives' confidentiality. They have not given permission and probably do not know that their details are being kept. This may be particularly relevant if there is an inherited genetic disease, for example. On the other hand, a family history is important for the diagnosis and treatment of the patient.

Reality TV and children

The vogue for reality TV programmes about childrens' hospitals has raised an important issue of confidentiality. Even though the parents of children and babies may have given permission for the film to be shown, the children may view it very differently when they grow up and find the whole country knows about their past medical history. Could this be an unjustified breach of the child's confidentiality, as it is clearly not in his or her best interest?

Telling children's parents

A difficult issue for many years has been the keeping of confidentiality of Gillick-competent children from their parents. In Chapter 7 we discussed how an under-age child can give consent for treatment but may not refuse life-saving therapy. Here we are concerned with a girl, say of 13, who wishes to go on the pill or is pregnant but does not want her parents to know. Is the doctor obliged to tell the parents or even the police, because having sex with a girl under 16 is 'statutory rape'? By failing to report it, the doctor would be condoning or encouraging a crime. Current Department of Health guidelines stress the importance of confidentiality for the under-16s (DH, 2004) but there is a suggestion that this may soon change.

The future

With genetic testing becoming more routine and more predictive of future illness, there will be increasing pressure on doctors to divulge details to life insurance companies. This particularly sensitive information should only be released with the patient's consent but one can foresee insurance companies or some employers refusing to take on patients who insist on their confidentiality. At present insurance companies in the UK have agreed with the Government to postpone the use of predictive genetic testing results until 2011.

Summary

- Confidentiality is fundamental to the trust between doctor and patient and must be protected.
- It is very easy to break patients' confidences unintentionally by chatting in the lift or corridor, on the telephone or by leaving notes where they can be easily seen.
- There are some clear situations where a doctor should break confidences by law.
- There are a few issues not yet resolved.
- The Data Protection Act 1998 has brought in new safeguards for written patient records.
- Obtaining the patient's consent is the most important safeguard of confidentiality.
- Relatives should not be given details without the patient's permission, except in special circumstances and only in the patient's best interest.
- Doctors do not have the right to see a friend's records, just because they are doctors.

10

JUSTICE AND FAIRNESS

In 1997, the *Lancet* carried a leader entitled 'Health inequality: the UK's biggest issue' (Editorial, 1997). It quoted from the original 1942 Beveridge Report (which was the blueprint for the National Health Service): 'a health service providing full preventive and curative treatment of every kind to every citizen without exceptions, without remuneration limit and without an economic barrier at any point to delay recourse to it, is the ideal plan'. This was a fine ideal but probably never realistic: because Beveridge did not foresee the huge and expensive advances in treatment, nor the effect of people living far longer as health care improved. More than 60 years later, today's UK Government is dedicated to abolishing so-called 'postcode prescribing', (where people in one area of the UK can obtain certain drugs or treatments but those in another area cannot). Sadly, there is a clear link between social deprivation and health and life expectancy.

Most people have a strong sense of natural justice and fairness, particularly when they concern the essentials of life such as food, warmth and health and when they are in short supply: this is termed distributive justice. During the Second World War in the UK all essentials such as food, clothes and petrol were rationed. The food ration was brilliantly planned to give

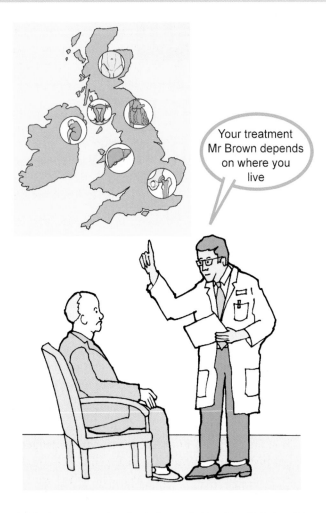

everybody just enough of a balanced diet. Implicit in this process was the idea that, even if you would like to have more than one egg per week, you went without the extra so that others could have the minimum. There was hardly any obesity and it has been said that the nation has never been healthier!

Governments running a national health service cannot **guarantee** people's health, because patients may not want to take advice or take advantage of particular treatments on offer. However, they can try to guarantee **access** to health care for everyone. This is a challenge even in wealthy Western democracies; but when the idea of justice is extended to developing countries world-wide, the challenge takes on a whole new dimension.

There are naturally emotional reactions to any idea of rationing health care, even though it has been implicit for years and has been renamed 'prioritization'. Len and Lesley Doyal have argued convincingly that the concept of rationing is not incompatible with the moral foundation of the National Health Service as conceived by Beveridge, but that the way it is carried out is critical (Doyal and Doyal, 1999).

WHY JUSTICE?

The whole idea of justice comes from a particular view of people – that they are all of equal worth and have equal rights. This does not mean they are equal in all ways. To many faith groups, the concept of justice assumes there is an 'ultimate judge'. As we have seen in Chapter 4, justice does not underlie all philosophies, religious or secular. The Hindu caste system or the Nazi philosophy of race do not pretend that people of different social or racial origins are of equal worth. Even superficially Christian Victorian England, which acknowledged the principles of justice and fairness, needed people who really took justice seriously. This is well illustrated by the work of people such as William Wilberforce, who abolished the slave trade, and Lord Shaftesbury and Dr Barnardo, who championed the rights of children.

Unselfishness

A National Health System needs an extraordinary degree of insight and unselfishness from the population. The very idea that we should pay a compulsory tax for the benefit of others is quite profound. Many other societies would not accept it especially when 'our' money is going to help people who have brought illness on themselves by their lifestyle.

Equity not equality

Fairness does not mean that everybody gets the same share, any more than food rationing gave to children or nursing mothers the same rations as men. Fairness, at its least, means that those with a similar condition and in the same circumstances get the same treatment and those with equal need receive equal care. The real problem comes when comparing treatments for different conditions in different people. How can they be evaluated?

PRIORITIZATION: ON WHAT CRITERIA?

The simplistic answer to problems of distributing scarce resources is to give a little to everyone. However, that might result in benefit to nobody. A small, ineffective dose of antibiotics to each of a group of people with pneumonia would not help, in the same way that giving too little food to each of a group of stranded sailors on a desert island would not save any lives. When scarce resources have to be shared out there has to be a priority order. The question is how can we decide? Box 10.1 shows some possible criteria that can be used.

Box 10.1   Possible criteria for prioritization

- Age
- Type of illness
- Merit – usefulness to society
- Demand – pressure groups
- Effectiveness of treatment
- Need.

Age

'Anti-ageism' is the current focus of political correctness and, indeed, the elderly are one of the Government priorities in health care. However, there has been a strong strand of thinking over the years that priority should be given to children and young people, because they stand to benefit more and should be helped to reach the age that the elderly have already reached. Age can never be a criterion in isolation, without considering the effectiveness of treatment and other factors. In the past, there has been an upper age cut-off for major treatments such as transplantation. This may be justified if the elderly have other co-morbidities that make the treatment less effective or more dangerous, but not just because of their age.

It is interesting to note how the upper limit of age for operations such as ruptured aneurysm and coronary artery bypass graft – or even dialysis – have crept up over the years as average life expectancy has increased (or as doctors making the decisions themselves become older!).

Type of illness

This criterion asserts that there are some conditions that are more important to treat than others. To put it at its simplest, everyone would agree that an operation for curable cancer should have priority over an operation for an in-growing toe-nail, or that the man with a sprained ankle should wait for his X-ray when the victims of a serious road accident are rushed into the A&E department. Along these lines we could draw up a simple list of priorities for category of disease:

1. Acute, life-threatening
2. Severe, chronic debilitating
3. Non-life-threatening, distressing
4. Minor, self-limiting.

This would probably gain general acceptance, although if money was so short that the third or fourth categories were never treated there would soon be rumblings of discontent. In practice, in the UK, the last category of illnesses are treated more and more by the patient themselves, by pharmacies and by complementary therapists.

Rationing so far in the NHS has been by waiting lists rather than a complete ban: a patient with suspected cancer is seen in the clinic within two weeks, whereas a patient with a mild skin condition may have to wait for months.

The Oregon example

The Health Service Commissioners of the state of Oregon in the USA have undertaken an interesting experiment in priority. They consulted members of the public as well as doctors, nurses and care workers of all kinds, to make a list of conditions and treatments in order of importance – a Prioritized List of Health Services (Oregon Health Services Commission, 2006). They then agreed to finance all treatments above a certain number in the table each year, the remainder not being eligible for State funding. Each year alterations and adaptations are made and in 2006 they financed from 1 to 530 out of a list of 710. At the top of the list were severe/moderate head injury, insulin-dependent diabetes and acute peritonitis and at the bottom benign conditions such as common cold and sebaceous cysts or conditions where there is no effective treatment. This priority list has been in use now for many years. The great advantage of such a mechanism is that the prioritization is transparent and the public can influence the order, and new treatments can also be added.

Demand

In a democracy, governments are influenced by public opinion and persistent lobbying by 'interest groups'. It is easy for those who shout loudest to gain a larger share of the economic cake. Thus diseases with strong Patient Associations and pressure groups may be given a disproportionally higher priority. However, recently the UK Department of Health has attempted to target the 'less attractive' conditions and those with low profile, such as mental health. Children with heart problems and malignant disease will always have more emotional appeal than the elderly with Alzheimer's disease: planners must not merely respond to publicity and emotive stories if they are to exercise justice.

Merit

It can be argued that those who put most into society should be the first to benefit from health finances, and consequently be kept healthy for the benefit of all. Kant thought that goods should be distributed according to the moral worth of people, not distributed equally. The Communist philosophy is that the military and factory workers are treated before the unemployed and retired. In the UK during the Second World War, penicillin was only produced in small quantities. It was given first to Winston Churchill, the Prime Minister, when he had pneumonia and then to the troops for war injuries. As it happens, the senior author of this book had a severe septicaemia in 1944 but was low down the priority list to receive the scarce new antibiotic; fortunately he survived to be able to tell the tale! In unusual times, such as wars, usefulness to the nation might be an appropriate criterion for priority, but not one that should be applied indiscriminately in peacetime.

Traditionally we do not exclude from treatment those who bring illness on themselves, but as the pressure on resources increases this has to be considered. For example the decision not to do a liver transplant for a patient with alcoholic cirrhosis and who has not stopped drinking is based more on effective-ness (the new liver will soon be damaged itself) rather than vindictiveness. Even if a patient has stopped drinking before a liver transplant, there is no guarantee they will not start again as the late footballer George Best sadly demonstrated. It is interesting that in the Oregon Prioritized List of Services conditions that are considered to be self-induced are given a relatively low priority despite their potential life-threatening consequences (Oregon Health Services Commission, 2006).

Effectiveness of treatments

Efficacy means that a treatment works under ideal conditions, whereas effectiveness means that it works when it is applied generally to the relevant population. For example, impaired effectiveness is one of the reasons for not doing cardiovascular surgery on people who continue to smoke even though the efficacy of these treatments has been shown beyond doubt. Cost effectiveness (also known as cost benefit or efficiency) means that a treatment is worth using. How can the effectiveness of different treatments for different patients be compared? Once a new drug is found to have efficacy, how can we know if it will be cost effective?

It was to answer these questions that health economists came up with the idea of quality-adjusted life years (QALYs) (Phillips and Thompson, 2001). Rather than just measure the prolongation of life in years, the quality of that life (QoL) is also measured 'by consideration of objectively and subjectively indicated well being in multiple domains of life considered salient in one's culture and time, while adhering to universal standards of human rights' (Koot, 2001). A figure of £20 000 per QALY has been suggested as an arbitrary cut-off point between what is cost-effective and what is not cost-effective. There has been much discussion of QALYs and their use; some of the arguments for and against are listed in Box 10.2. Of particular concern is the group of patients who have less potential for improvement and will always score poorly, whichever measurement is used ('double jeopardy') (Harris, 1995).

Box 10.2   Assessment of QALYs

In favour

- They take a holistic view of the quality of a patient's life
- In practice they have been used to inform rather than dictate funding decisions
- They consider both quality and quantity of life
- We cannot ignore the cost of treatment and it would be unfair just to make decisions on guesswork

- The £20 000 cut-off is just a guide and not sacrosanct
- They expose highly expensive and ineffective treatments.

Criticisms

- They may confuse quality of life with a person's value (see Chapter 4)
- They are utilitarian in philosophy (see Chapter 3)
- When patients are already handicapped there is less chance of improving their quality of life so they may miss out ('double jeopardy')
- The arbitrary cut-off at £20 000 per QALY leads to inequity
- They may ignore individual patient's wishes because they are based on standard questionnaires.

Another problem is that QALYs are based on patient groups and the evidence is mainly derived from controlled trials, which may not be representative. Individuals have different ambitions and respond differently to the same intervention. A new drug is licensed on the basis of efficacy and safety. In the UK, the National Institute for Health and Clinical Excellence (NICE) evaluates a large range of health interventions and issues guidelines on effective and cost-effectiveness and which patients will benefit. In practice NICE uses QALYs as only one factor of their overall assessment, and an expensive treatment for a rare and serious condition is given special consideration and not just ignored because it has a high cost per QALY.

Futile and ineffective treatments

One thing is clear in all this discussion: it is wasteful and unethical to use expensive treatments that do not work or have only minimal effects. Yet there is strong emotional pressure on doctors (from themselves and from patients' relatives) to 'do something'.

Need

An alternative to prioritizing by demand or merit is by **need**; those whose needs are greatest have priority. Needs may be financial or social in addition to medical. It has been said that the test of a civilized society is the way it treats its poorest citizens. Care and social reforms in the nineteenth century and the health reform of the twentieth century in the UK have taken seriously the Christian commitment to the poor and those unable to help themselves. In so doing they followed the example of the monasteries of the middle ages. In the USA, State medical services have special arrangements through Medicare and Medicaid for vulnerable groups.

Need must also include a patient's responsibility for dependants – whether old or young: a single mother with three young children might be given priority over a retired woman with no dependants with the same illness.

From a world-wide perspective, if need is the criterion, most of the world's medical resources should be directed to the developing countries of Africa and Asia. Pressure from individuals and organizations is having an effect on Western governments. When there is an appeal for aid after a disaster, tsunami or earthquake, the public response is huge, based on compassion, need and justice.

PREVENTION VERSUS TREATMENT

One of the most difficult problems in the fair distribution of resources is how to balance short-term treatments with prevention of future illness. When there is an immediate important need it is difficult to earmark money to prevent future illnesses that have not yet happened! Yet prevention is often cheap, simple and cost-effective, although the financial benefits are often not seen for many years. The immunization programme for children, for example, has produced huge benefits, including the abolition or virtual abolition of both smallpox and polio from the world. But when a vaccine becomes available for the human immunodeficiency virus (HIV), should priority go to immunizing those who do not yet have the infection or treating those who are already suffering? Ideally, we should do both, but it is easy in the current atmosphere of short-term financial accounting to give prevention a low priority. On the other hand, 10 years ago who would have imagined that Parliament would vote on a total smoking ban in public places, even though the cost is transferred to the pub landlord!

THRESHOLDS FOR TREATMENT

When chronic illnesses are very common, the threshold for treatment can vary greatly from doctor to doctor and place to place. This can have a huge effect on costs. For example, a large number of people over 50 suffer from some degree of hypertension. At what level of blood pressure should treatment start? There are now some guidelines for this. Similarly a large proportion have a raised cholesterol level: at what level should treatment start? (see Chapter 12).

Guidelines may change. Some degree of osteoarthritis of the hip affects the majority of people over 65, giving variable amounts of pain. What level of pain or X-ray changes make the surgeon decide to operate? The lowering of the threshold (which is not yet agreed) would put thousands more people on the waiting list every year, at significant cost.

There is a pressing need for agreement between health managers, patients and doctors on thresholds for intervention in many of the common medical and surgical conditions. In the interests of justice, decisions must be made, even though patients below the threshold will continue to suffer from discomfort and some risk.

There is a school of thought that claims it is unfair to give a treatment to **anybody** if it cannot be given to **everybody**. This would certainly stop the development of new treatments and hardly support the obligation to do good!

PRIVATE PRACTICE

The issue of private practice in the UK produces strong emotions, and cries are heard of 'Queue-jumping', 'One system for the rich and another for the poor', 'Surgeons keep long waiting lists to fuel their private practice'. There is nothing intrinsically unethical about a private health system, especially if it is financed by private insurance, provided there is a safety net for those who genuinely cannot afford it. The problems arise when a private and a public system run in parallel and the same doctors work in both. Doctors have to be very careful that there is not a conflict of interests, and that private practice does not set the agenda or decisions for the public health system.

In the UK patients with private means or insurance can 'jump the queue' but some justice is preserved, because they continue to pay their NHS contributions: in effect they pay twice. Ideally, the waiting lists should be short enough so that queue-jumping is not an issue. Then private medicine would be comparable with buying a first class ticket on the train – the first-class passenger gets more comfort, but the same driver is taking all passengers to the same destination at the same time.

Top-up fees

An alternative strategy, which has been applied to dental care, is to provide a standard cost-effective treatment in the public system and let those who wish to have gold fillings pay the extra. This could be applied to joint replacement in orthopaedics where there is a wide range of costs. In the past, wards had single side rooms known as 'amenity beds' which patients could book for a supplementary payment, but this did not mean that they were queue-jumping. The condition was also that the room would be given up if a very sick patient needed it.

CONCLUSION: TRANSPARENCY

Clearly one single criterion is inadequate to make the difficult decisions about fair distribution of medical resources (equity). Need must be balanced by effectiveness, and demand by cost-effectiveness. The concept of priority (rationing) will only be accepted by a population if it knows and understands the criteria, however imperfect, on which the decisions have been based. Throughout the process there must also be willingness to consider the needs of others. Oregon paved the way for transparency and other systems are following, but this involves extensive consultation and explanation to the 'healthy' public and the many patient groups. If, as a society, we think that it is an ethical imperative to spread health care fairly, and particularly help those in the lower socio-economic groups, we need to have sound methods as well as pious hopes.

Summary

- Justice and equity are important ethical principles.
- The concept of fairness arises from the concept of equal intrinsic value of all human beings.
- There is significant inequality within developed countries, and extreme inequality around the world.
- Rationing or prioritization cannot be avoided, even in the most developed country.
- Rationing may be based on age, type of illness, merit, demand, (cost-)effectiveness or need.
- Need should be the primary consideration, but must be informed by other criteria.
- The process must be transparent, consistent and evidence-based.

11

TRUTH AND INTEGRITY

It is curious that major ethical codes such as the Hippocratic Oath and the Declaration of Geneva say nothing about an 'obligation to truthfulness', and some books on medical ethics do not even have these words in their index. Is it just assumed? As we have already mentioned, 40 years ago it was quite common for a doctor to lie to a patient about a diagnosis of cancer, or, at least, to use medical phrases that concealed the truth (e.g. 'It's not cancer; it's a type of tumour'). This was done with the best of intentions, to try to spare the patient's distress, but the same doctors would have been furious if the same patient had lied to them. Of course malignant tumours vary widely in their rate of growth and their prognosis, so, it was argued, the word 'cancer' could give quite the wrong impression if used for a very slow growing tumour because the word to many people immediately implies a painful and lingering death.

There is a world of difference between trying to conceal or distort the truth on the one hand, and using less frightening words that the patient understands and which convey the right impression, on the other. It is possible to speak the truth but convey nothing to the patient. Over the last 40 years there has been a large and welcome change in attitudes to patients knowing about their own diseases. This is partly due to the influence of the hospice movement. But, as in many situations, there is a danger of the pendulum swinging too far and the reaction against concealing the truth to spare the patients' distress may become the blunt and unsympathetic unloading of all the facts at once onto vulnerable anxious people. Although truth is not especially stated in some codes, the General Medical Council (GMC) list of duties of a doctor includes 'Being honest and trustworthy; acting with integrity' (GMC, 2001). In addition to when it comes to research, the Declaration of Helsinki is adamant that subjects should be told all the known risks. Without truthfulness there can be no real doctor/patient relationship or meaningful ethical debate.

WHAT IS TRUTH?

This is one of the key philosophical questions that has been asked down the ages. The whole of the medical and research enterprise is based on the assumption that there is an objective truth to find – that there are such diseases as gallstones, cancer, osteoarthritis that can be identified and agreed among pathologists world-wide. However, no scientist would claim that we know **all** the truth and wise scientists recognize their own biases and emotional involvement and must come to terms with the fact that their theories may be proved wrong.

> *'The great tragedy of science – the slaying of a beautiful hypothesis by an ugly fact'* wrote TH Huxley.
> (Huxley HA, 1907)

In medicine, we have to live with uncertainty and must often make decisions with inadequate information.

Modernists and post-modernists have very different attitudes from the traditional view of truth. They argue that truth is not something objective that we can all agree on, but rather something that may be true for one person and not for another or that only becomes true if I say it is.

These differences can be illustrated by three football referees debating their attitude to goal-line decisions (adapted from

Guinness, 2000). The first says 'The ball has either crossed the line or it has not, and my decision reflects what actually happened.' He represents the traditional view of truth. The second says: 'That is arrogant; the ball may or may not have crossed the line, but I base my decision on how I see it.' He represents modern relativism. The third says: 'It may or may not have crossed the line, but it is not a goal until I say it is.' He represents post-modernism.

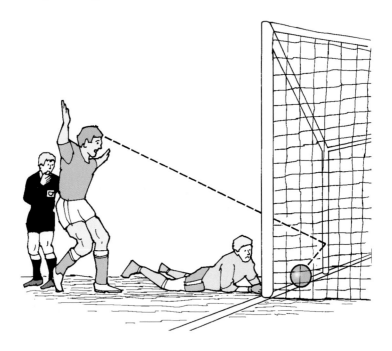

Judging by the frequent calls for television replays and supporters' cries of 'We've been robbed!', the vast football-viewing public clearly believes in the first view of truth!

Historically, from the ancient Greeks onwards, truth has been linked with freedom. Attitudes to truth illustrate very well the differences between the ethical theories described in Chapter 3 and the different value systems discussed in Chapter 4. To a deontologist, especially one with a religious value system, speaking the truth is a fundamental duty which should be obeyed (except in exceptional circumstances) irrespective of the consequences. The whole legal system is based on a witness swearing 'to speak the truth, the whole truth and nothing but the truth', and interestingly, the Bible is still used as the guarantee of the authority of that statement in the UK. However, to a utilitarian, speaking the truth is judged by its results – whether it produces happiness or not. The truth may produce initial unhappiness but satisfaction later on, whereas a lie has the reverse effect. To the atheistic Darwinian, truth is unnecessary and often an encumbrance. John Gray states 'Darwinian theory tells us that an interest in truth is not needed for survival or reproduction. ... In a competition for mates a well developed capacity for self deception is an advantage' (Gray, 2002, page 27)!

Medicine, science and practice must rest on the assumption that there is objective medical truth that is discoverable, yet partial. Moreover without that connection medical research is aimless. However, any doctor must hold knowledge with humility, knowing that new knowledge may change treatment and we must all be prepared to admit ignorance – a task made more difficult by the media spin and hype that greets each new discovery.

A simple example is the diet for patients with diverticular disease. Forty years ago it was thought (on not very strong evidence) that a high-roughage diet was responsible for the diverticula, so patients were advised to have a low-roughage diet. Thirty years ago research revealed that a low-residue diet produced slow bowel transit, constipation and high intracolonic pressure, so the advice was completely reversed and patients put on a high-residue diet!

Another example is the recent change in understanding of the causes of peptic ulcers. Twenty years ago, a student suggesting in an exam that ulcers should be treated with antibiotics would have failed!

We must now ask some questions about truth in practice.

TELLING PATIENTS THE TRUTH

There is an unwritten contract of trust between doctor and patient which demands honesty from both sides: if a doctor decides to deceive, trust is lost. Moreover, patients cannot exercise their autonomy without knowing the facts.

What should we tell patients?

It is sometimes difficult to give information that is specific for an individual. Our knowledge of prognosis is statistical, with a median and range for a population with that particular disease. The range is often wide and we may not know where on the graph any particular patient lies. So to say to a patient 'The survival for your condition is between six months and two years' is not being evasive but far more truthful than saying 'You have nine months to live' (a phrase, by the way, that is often quoted but hardly ever said!). However, the most important aspect is to allow patients to ask the questions that they want to ask and to answer them as honestly as possible, including admitting 'I don't know'.

What if the patient does not want to know?

Patients have a perfect right **not** to know, in the same way as they have a perfect right to refuse treatment, but they cannot exercise both rights at the same time. Sometimes there is an opportunity, before a diagnosis is made, to come to an arrangement. For example, before an operation, when the diagnosis is not clear, a surgeon might ask the patient how much he or she wants to know about the findings. The patient may want to be told everything or reply 'Just fix it but don't bother me about the details'. However there are times when it is in the patient's best interest to be told, even if he or she appears not to want to know the truth. For example, a patient may be starting a new business deal in the near future or planning to go to see a new grand-daughter in Australia next year. The gentle advice 'I would go sooner rather than later' may be needed.

How to tell the truth – breaking bad news

Any doctor, however experienced, who finds it easy to break bad news has lost all compassion and sensitivity; but a doctor who cannot handle a patient's emotions, and so avoids facing the issue is equally unhelpful. How often do we hear the remark 'The patient reacted badly to the news of her diagnosis'? which usually means she was shocked and burst into tears. But that reaction may not be bad for the patient; suppressing a natural response may lead to more serious emotional problems later. It is important not to take away hope – but it must be a realistic hope. 'We will soon have you up and about' can sound trite and is probably not true. But 'There is nothing more we can do' is never true. A change from a curative aim to symptom relief (palliation) can be very positive.

The clues to imparting the unpleasant truth are sensitivity and timing. Most patients cannot take everything in at once, and need the time to think about the initial information and decide which further questions to ask. The non-paternalistic doctor is there to share information with the patient, not to give doctor's orders or doctor's opinions when not requested. Some information can be conveyed without words and understanding reached without the use of painful words such as cancer, but this concept is often wishful thinking. There are many occasions when the plain question 'Is it cancer doctor?' cannot be avoided.

A patient visiting the USA for a conference developed obstructive jaundice. He was operated on and found to have a lump in his pancreas, which was thought to be a cancer obstructing his bile duct and an operation to bypass it was performed. Unusually, for the USA, he was told that there was no cancer, but his wife was told the 'true' diagnosis. He could not understand why his wife was so sad. He came to England and obtained a second opinion because he was still jaundiced. A re-operation found that the cause of the jaundice was a gallstone which was also partly blocking the bypass and the lump in his pancreas was a

*benign cyst. Both were then told the truth. He was somewhat
puzzled that his wife was so overjoyed. The original surgeon had
thought he was telling the patient a lie, and his wife the truth,
when in fact it was the other way round!*

Giving information when there is a language barrier

When doctor and patient do not share a first language, the
doctor needs to make special arrangements. It should also be
remembered that there may be problems when the interpreter is
a family member but not next of kin. Most hospitals in the UK
have interpreters who are trained and respect confidentiality.

Talking with children

Although children may not be able to understand fully their
illness and treatment, this does **not** justify deception. Children
are often more perceptive than adults give them credit for and
part of any paediatric attachment is learning how to communi-
cate truthfully and appropriately with different aged children.
See Gillick competence p. 86.

Telling the truth when things go wrong

Doctors are human beings; human beings make mistakes.
However, if one has been made, the patient should be informed
of the problem, told how things can be put right, and reassured
that the cause will be investigated urgently and thoroughly.
Many complaints to hospitals and threatened legal actions arise
because a patient thinks that there has been a 'cover-up'. The
doctor's first responsibility is to tell the patient, not to appor-
tion nor prevent blame.

Gossip

Hospitals and medical schools are hotbeds of gossip. Whereas a
motto in the Second World War was 'Careless talk costs lives',

in modern practice, gossip can ruin careers! 'He is not a good operator' commented a senior consultant about a specialist registrar being considered for a surgical post. When asked if he had ever seen him operate, he had to admit, with embarrassment, that he had not. Criticizing colleagues' actions to patients is hardly every justified; moreover it is all too easy for a hospital consultant to criticize a GP's diagnosis two days before when the symptoms and signs were quite different.

INTEGRITY

The word 'integrity' comes from the Latin for 'soundness' or 'wholeness'. It involves sincerity, consistency, promise-keeping and not abusing your position as a doctor. 'Sincere' comes originally from a Greek word meaning 'without wax', because tradesman selling pottery would try to conceal cracks with wax. If a purchaser held the pot up to the sun, the crack could be seen! Hence it conveys the idea of not deceiving and not hiding flaws.

> *Integrity without knowledge is weak and useless. Knowledge without integrity is dangerous and dreadful.*
>
> (Samuel Johnson)

Research fraud

There has been a long history of deception in research, from the Piltdown Man hoax in 1912 to cloning and stem cell claims in South Korea in 2006. Plagiarism is an increasing problem.

Promise keeping

The most difficult promise to keep for the busy doctor is 'I will come back and discuss it with you in more detail later'. Sadly, all too often we hear a patient's resigned comment to her relatives

'He never did'. If we have forgotten, it is far better when coming back to say so rather than give a complicated explanation
about some emergency getting in the way. Similarly, if we
promise that we will not tell a patient's family something we
must honour that promise. Wise doctors are very careful not to
make promises they may not be able to keep. For discussion of
the student's dilemma see Chapter 15.

Integrity in relationships with patients

One of the key tenets of the ancient Hippocratic Oath is not
to abuse the special relationship between doctor and patient:
'Whatever houses I may visit, I will come for the benefit of the
sick, remaining free of all intentional injustice, of all mischief,
and in particular sexual relations with both female and male
persons, be they free or slaves' (Edelstein, 1943). Or, in the more
succinct words of the GMC: 'Never abuse your position as a
doctor' (GMC, 2001). Patients must be able to rely on their doctor's action and the boundaries of the professional relationship.

The abuse referred to by the GMC is not necessarily sexual; it
could equally be financial. For example, it could be considered
abusive for a doctor to recommend a private operation that is
not strictly necessary or to suggest that, if the patient paid to
go privately, the operation could be done next week.

Integrity in signing documents

Doctors often have to sign death certificates, cremation forms,
sickness notes, insurance reports and references for juniors for
job applications. It is so easy when you are busy to put your
signature to something that you have not personally checked. In
the days before self-certification for short-term sick leave, GPs
were sometimes put under great pressure to sign patients 'off
sick', when they knew perfectly well that they only had a slight
cold and wanted to watch the local football derby!

Indeed colleagues of Harold Shipman were criticized for not
checking more carefully before signing the second part of

cremation certificates. Fake CVs for job applications and not entirely accurate travel claims are being seen more often: it is a high-risk strategy, even for utilitarians!

Conflicts of interests

A few years ago, a Sunday newspaper checked on the shareholdings of members of two committees advising the UK Department of Health on licensing and appropriate use of new drugs. They discovered that several members had shares in major drug companies and others had received large drug firm grants for their research. However great these doctors' personal integrity, it is difficult to convince a sceptical public that they would not be biased when deciding which drugs to license and promote.

In recent years, many medical journals have insisted on a declaration of competing interests at the foot of each article, so that the reader can judge whether the article is biased. It is very difficult to avoid some conflicts of interest, but integrity is preserved by declaring it. Most drug trials are sponsored by the drug company concerned, but integrity is maintained by having independent statisticians and ethical advice. It can be embarrassing, even at a local meeting while discussing the addition of a new drug to the hospital pharmacy, to note that one of the members is using a pen with the company's name emblazoned on its side!

For British Members of Parliament the rules are clearly laid down by the Nolan Committee and these rules are adopted by all official committees. Entertainment by commercial companies must be appropriate and proportionate to the educational value of the event. A free skiing holiday with the occasional lecture in the evening does not fulfil this criterion. Because of abuse, the guidelines are being tightened all the time.

Occasional exceptions to truth telling are discussed in Chapter 12, but respecting the truth is fundamental to all ethical practice.

Summary

- Truth is the basis of trust between doctor and patient.
- Truth is fundamental to all aspects of ethical practice.
- Both clinical and research endeavours depend on the understanding that there is an objective truth that can be discovered.
- Modern and post-modern views make truth subjective.
- Utilitarians see truth an expendable means to an end.
- Unpleasant truth should be conveyed to patients gradually and sensitively.
- Patients have the right not to know the truth about their illness.
- Integrity means keeping promises, admitting mistakes and avoiding conflicts of interest.

12

COMPETING ETHICAL PRINCIPLES: DECIDING PRIORITIES

If there were no competition between different ethical obligations, there would be no ethical dilemmas and no need to write a book on the subject! Those who think there is no black and white but only shades of grey (see Chapter 2), imply that all principles have to be watered down and merged into one another, whereby each loses its distinctive quality. For example, to tell a half-truth in order to try to conserve partial confidentiality is unsatisfactory, and to give somebody partial autonomy so that we can treat them partly and do them some good honours neither principle.

A far more helpful concept is that good principles may compete and we have to decide which has priority or carries more weight in a particular situation. This does not mean that one or other is ignored, but one is temporarily made less important. However, it must always be restored to its rightful place before further decisions are made. Often it is possible to honour both or all ethical principles by the way we handle the dilemmas – the way we explain things to patients or the way we devise the details of research projects.

Figure 12.1 illustrates the different options available when two ethical principles are competing, while Figure 12.2 puts this into a medical context.

LESSER OF TWO EVILS

Typically the expression 'lesser of two evils' is used for such situations as a young teenage girl becoming pregnant as a result of rape, where neither abortion nor continuing with the pregnancy is ideal ('good') and therefore both options might be considered 'evil'. The argument can be reversed by saying it is good to preserve the foetus and good to preserve the physical and mental health of the teenage mother, but it may not be possible to do both 'goods'. However, as in other dilemmas, by careful management it may be possible to do both. It is important to note that by definition no ethical dilemma in the health field starts from an ideal position because the patient already has a problem; but it is equally important to remember that if a doctor has to decide on the 'lesser of two evils', that does not make it good: it is still far from ideal either to destroy the foetus or damage the girl's mental health and development.

PRIORITY OF ETHICAL PRINCIPLES

From previous chapters we have found that there is general agreement about the following five ethical principles (in alphabetical order):

Box 12.1   Alphabetical order
1. Autonomy and consent
2. Beneficence and non-maleficence
3. Confidentiality
4. Justice and equity
5. Truth and integrity.

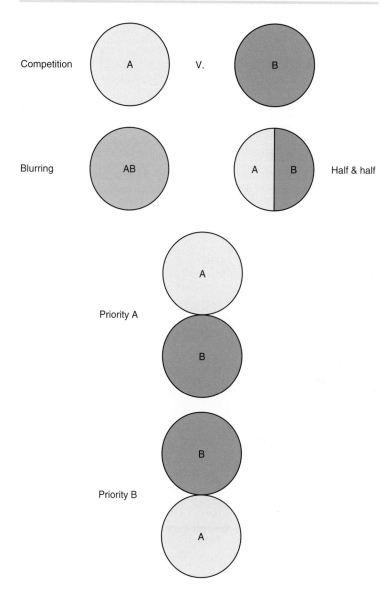

Figure 12.1 Options when two ethical principles are competing

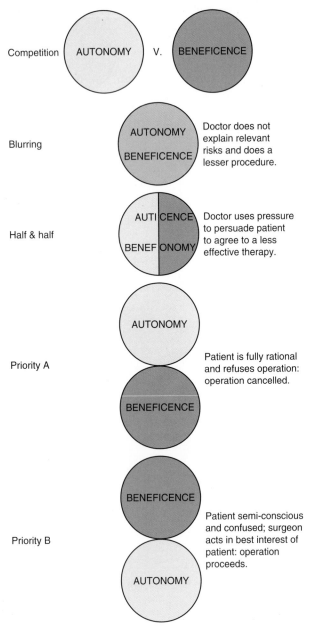

Figure 12.2 Options when there is a possibility of a patient refusing an operation that could be of great benefit

It could be argued that confidentiality and consent are both parts of autonomy (see Chapters 7 and 9) but they do sometimes compete with each other, so, for the moment, it will be helpful to consider them separately. The key question is whether this list represents the correct priority order of these principles when applied to a clinical situation. For example, should autonomy always have preference over doing good to the patient or over justice for other people? As discussed in Chapter 7 this is an extreme view of autonomy. This order also assumes that doing good should always have priority over confidentiality, so that if we can help a patient by breaking confidence that is justified. Finally, if we put truth and integrity at the bottom, telling lies or half-truths can always be justified if it benefits the patient or keeps confidentiality.

From the purely **ethical**, as opposed to **legal**, perspective the following priority order could be justified:

Box 12.2   Ethical priority order

1. Truth and integrity
2. Beneficence and non-maleficence
3. Justice and fairness
4. Autonomy and consent
5. Confidentiality.

We have argued in Chapter 11 that without truth and integrity all ethical systems collapse, because if a patient does not tell the doctor the truth about his or her illness and the doctor does not keep faith with the patient, then the other principles cannot work in practice. Justice depends on integrity and honesty about the real situation. The patient who does not trust the doctor to tell the truth about the benefits and risks of an operation is not going to give consent. Justice is put above autonomy because justice cannot happen if autonomy is dominant, and autonomy can turn into selfishness, which does not take into account other people's needs.

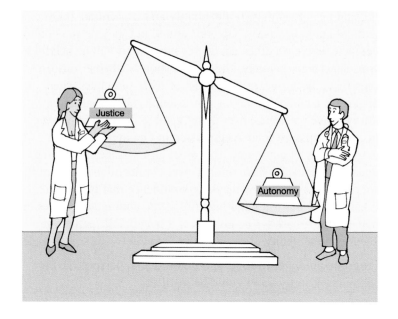

From the current **legal** perspective on the other hand, the order of priority is as follows:

Box 12.3   Legal priority order

1. Autonomy
2. Beneficence and non-maleficence
3. Confidentiality
4. Truth and integrity
5. Justice and fairness.

There is a strong move to give justice a higher priority in the UK and also in other parts of the world where the inequalities may be far greater. Under English law patients have the right to refuse treatment that may benefit them. In a number of situations truth is subjugated to political correctness and health workers are not free to describe the real situation.

Whichever priority order is adopted, there are occasions when something lower in the priority order has to be brought higher, but that does not mean that it should always stay in that position, unless it is important also on other occasions. A series of clinical examples will help us to understand how the competition between these principles occurs and how it can be handled. All these examples are real, not hypothetical, although one or two details have been altered.

TRUTH VERSUS BENEFICENCE

A 55-year-old woman has come into hospital for investigations for anaemia and shortness of breath. She says she will kill herself if she is found to have cancer. The results confirm a malignant tumour. Do you risk her life by telling her she has cancer?

Assuming you are fairly sure she will carry out her threat, you have to decide whether to honour the truth at all costs over the value of her life, or intentionally deceive her in order to preserve her life (beneficence). As mentioned in Chapter 11, telling lies to patients with cancer was standard practice for many years in the last century and often the justification for it was that the doctor had heard of a patient who had committed suicide after being told the diagnosis. This illustrates well that if in an exceptional circumstance, with a particularly anxious patient, the doctor decides that not telling the whole truth is justified, it must **not** become a normal practice as it did for 50 years. In reality, skilful questioning and finding out what she understands by cancer and enabling her come to terms with her illness gradually can honour both ethical principles and in the end do her far more good than a 'quick lie' that has to be unravelled, with difficulty, later – and may have far-reaching consequences for the patient's and her relatives' trust in the doctor.

TRUTH VERSUS CONFIDENTIALITY

A 30-year-old man in a small four-bedded ward asks out loud whether his HIV test was positive. Just before the ward round started the team had received the result, which is positive. Do you answer truthfully and therefore risk the rest of the ward knowing, by breaking confidentiality, or do you tell a lie and then explain to him afterwards that you did so to protect his confidentiality?

According to purely ethical priorities (Box 12.2, page 139) you should tell him the truth because this has priority over confidentiality. But from a legal perspective you should preserve confidentiality by any means necessary. It might seem easy just to say 'I will tell you afterwards' but that would always be interpreted as meaning it is positive. If you whisper, the rest of the ward will assume a positive result. In this particular case, the right course of action is clearer: by asking out loud, knowing others could hear, the patient had already himself broken confidentiality and therefore has given you the right to answer truthfully, although of course you would do so as discretely as possible, trying to avoid other people overhearing. Discussing confidential details in an open ward is particularly difficult if the patient is hard of hearing.

AUTONOMY VERSUS BENEFICENCE

A frightened 60-year-old woman is seen in the clinic and the doctor advises her that she should have a mastectomy for cancer of the breast and that there is a fair chance of curing it. After the details are explained to her she refuses the operation and says she is going to see a friend of hers who is a hypnotherapist. How can you protect her from possible harm while honouring her autonomy?

Under present UK law there is nothing you can do to enforce a beneficial operation on an unwilling patient, provided that you are satisfied that she is completely rational and understands the consequences of her refusal. Autonomy takes priority over beneficence (Box 12.3, page 140). However, this example also shows that a decision can be reversible. You can maintain the possibility of beneficence by your attitude. Instead of being affronted and react by saying 'Oh well if you do not want my advice I am no longer prepared to take care of you', you could offer help by saying 'If, after a time, you decide that you want to come back to me, I will be only too willing to try to help you further'. You could also give a further clinic appointment and advise her to discuss it with her GP. It may be tempting to find her relatives and ask them to persuade her to have an operation, but that would add a further problem by breaching the ethical principle of confidentiality.

BENEIFICENCE VERSUS AUTONOMY

A 26-year-old man comes into the A&E department after a motorcycle accident smelling of alcohol. He is semi-conscious from a head injury but also has evidence of intra-abdominal bleeding and needs an urgent, probably life-saving, operation. How can you save his life and respect his autonomy?

It is an important ethical imperative to do good (beneficence) but also important to have consent to preserve the patient's autonomy. You could wait for the patient's consciousness to improve to obtain consent, but that might be too late. Clearly in this situation the duty to save his life takes precedence over the need to get valid consent, even if later it transpires that he crashed his motorcycle on purpose in order to commit suicide. Trying to blend the two ethical principles and have a bit of consent and a bit of beneficence would obviously achieve nothing. The law will uphold your course of action on the reasonable assumption that he would have wished to be treated, even though autonomy has top priority in legal terms (Box 12.3, page 140).

BENIFICENCE VERSUS AUTONOMY AND JUSTICE INVOLVING MORE THAN ONE PERSON

Example 1

A white male kidney donor leaves his kidney for transplantation after his death on condition it is only given to a white recipient. If you were the transplant surgeon, would you accept it?

In this example, there is clear competition between doing good to a white patient (beneficence) on the one hand, and lack of justice, on the other, in that a patient could be denied a kidney transplantation because of the colour of his or her skin. To refuse to accept the kidney at all would mean no one would benefit. The order of priority in both ethical and legal terms would suggest that the transplantation should go ahead to benefit at least one person. Most people's instinctive reaction would suggest that justice should be placed higher up the priority order and the kidney should be refused, but is this just an emotional response? An alternative course of action to maintain beneficence and justice is to ignore the donor's autonomy and go ahead and transplant the patient with the best tissue match whatever their skin colour. This might be the right ethical action but would have legal consequences and there is no time for a long legal discussion, which would delay the operation and increase the risk that the transplanted kidney would fail.

Example 2

A 30-year-old woman refuses a caesarean section that would be essential to save the life of her normal full-term child. Can you compel her to have an operation? Is she rational to exercise her rights in this way?

This is a clear example of the competition between autonomy of the mother and the value and rights of the unborn child. The mother may well have been thinking of the very small risk to her life from the operation and so 'not doing harm' (non-maleficence) is also a consideration here. In this case, doctors had the patient admitted compulsorily to a psychiatric hospital ('sectioned') because they argued that such a decision implied that she was mentally unstable. Once she was in the hospital they operated on her without her consent. The law said that they were wrong on two counts. Consent is still required even for a patient who has been admitted compulsorily to a psychiatric hospital, if she can still understand the issues involved. Second, the unborn child, under UK law, has no rights. This may be the law, but is it ethical? If a parent refuses permission for life-saving treatment for her newborn child, the courts can overrule her to save the child. As we have seen in Chapter 4, there are now increasingly polarized attitudes to the rights of the newborn child as there have been for years to the rights of the unborn child.

BENEFICENCE VERSUS NON-MALEFICENCE (DOING GOOD VERSUS HARM)

A man needs coronary artery bypass surgery for severe angina but he is 75 and has diabetes. Can you ensure that the treatment will benefit him without doing harm?

There is a real opportunity to improve his life significantly but a 3–5 per cent risk of his dying as a result of the operation. Clearly the intention is to do good but there is a real risk of doing harm. This conflict is resolved by truth, autonomy and consent and that means giving the patient the facts in a way that he can understand and letting him take the decision. This, in a way, resolves the conflict for the surgeon and puts the responsibility back on to the patient.

Most medical and surgical treatments have side-effects and therefore pure beneficence is not possible. The more powerful the drug and the more serious the operation the higher the possibilities of both help and harm and all major operations carry a real but often very small mortality.

BENEFICENCE VERSUS NON-MALEFICENCE – MORE THAN ONE PERSON

A 16-year-old girl has severe diabetes and could benefit greatly in the long term from a pancreas transplant. Her mother offers to have part of her pancreas removed to transplant into her daughter. How can the surgeon do good to the patient without doing harm to her mother?

There is a risk to the operation of partial pancreatectomy but also a risk that the mother (donor) might become diabetic herself if too much of the pancreas is taken. As in previous examples, giving the mother the facts and not putting pressure on her helps to maintain her autonomy; but when family members are ill, emotions are strong and it is difficult to ensure objective informed consent.

The side-effects or possible harm are sometimes clearly known but often they are not and the consequences of treatment may not be foreseen. For example, the widespread use of the contraceptive pill, a great benefit to many women, has had the unforeseen side-effect of increasing exponentially the prevalence of sexually transmitted diseases. Although it was not the only cause of increased promiscuity, it enabled casual sex to be 'safe' from one 'side-effect' but not from others.

JUSTICE VERSUS INDIVIDUAL AUTONOMY

Example 1

In 1952 a new drug, streptomycin, was introduced in the USA for the treatment of tuberculosis (TB). Before that, the mainstay of treatment was fresh air and good food to try to help the body's own immune system to control the disease. However, in the UK only a relatively small quantity was available so there was not enough drug to treat all the patients. What should the doctors have done? How could they have prioritized patients for treatment while, at the same time, being fair?

The ethical principle of fairness and justice was being severely challenged in this situation. First they gave streptomycin to those with widespread (miliary) TB (i.e. the most severely ill with little chance of getting better spontaneously without direct treatment). By doing so they were not saying that these people were more valuable but, at the time, they were more needy (see Chapter 4). There were, however, no objective criteria by which priorities could be made for the rest.

In order to be fair, and not to select by subjective criteria such as age, good looks, social standing and usefulness to society, the treatment team decided to randomize, blindly, half the patients to receive the new treatment and half to continue on the fresh air regime. This had two results: firstly it showed conclusively that streptomycin was an effective treatment for TB and, secondly, it set the methodology for assessing all drugs in the future – the randomized, controlled trial.

Example 2

When new drugs came out for the lowering of cholesterol levels (statins) the Department of Health realized that if they were given to everybody with only a slightly raised cholesterol level, this one drug group would use up nearly all the total drug bill of the NHS. The Standing Medical Advisory Committee to the Secretary of State for Health, (SMAC) was asked for advice. How would you maintain justice by a fair plan of treatment?

A decision to give statins to the majority of those with raised cholesterol would deprive millions of other patients treatment for their different diseases. But once the benefits were known to the public, those with a raised cholesterol and therefore an increased risk of heart attack or stroke might exercise their autonomy and demand treatment. Here is clear competition between beneficence and the autonomy of some and the justice and fairness and the value of other people's lives. In the event, SMAC advised the drug should be given to those with the greatest risk and the threshold was a 3 per cent risk of a stroke or heart attack in the following year, based on a risk assessment which included hypertension, smoking and diabetes. At that time even this decision meant spending £250 million a year on statins. Judgement therefore was made on severity of risk and maximizing the benefit to some and denying a slighter benefit to others.

This introduces another autonomy issue: should those who continue to smoke and exercise their autonomy in this way and increase their risk be given the benefit of expensive drugs.

> To attempt to honour both beneficence and justice by giving a small dose of a drug to everybody would satisfy neither.

AUTONOMY AND CONFIDENTIALITY VERSUS JUSTICE

In 2002 there was an epidemic of severe acute respiratory syndrome (SARS) in Asia. Patients' rights to travel were withdrawn and they were stopped and questioned at airports in order to prevent a world-wide epidemic. Was it justified to infringe individual autonomy for the sake of others?

This restriction of autonomy was generally accepted internationally. It is accepted in the UK that certain infectious diseases should be reported to the Health Authorities to limit their spread and reduce the dangers to others. This involves breaking confidentiality. In the past, patients with disease such as smallpox and tuberculosis were detained compulsorily in isolation hospitals, thereby restricting autonomy in the interest of justice for others.

It is fascinating to see the very different ethical stance over HIV/AIDS. When faced with the most serious world epidemic for many years, 'authorities' have decided that confidentiality and individual autonomy should be given priority over the safety of others so that patients' cannot be tested against their will and there is no restriction on their behaviour (see Chapter 14). The authorities justify this difference from the management of SARS by pointing out that to acquire HIV needs a conscious action on the part of the person whereas SARS can be caught accidentally by just being close to a person in an aeroplane. Is such a distinction justified? Why should a doctor be accused of intruding in a patient's autonomy by recommending a change in sexual behaviour whereas it is quite acceptable to advise a change in lifestyle for smoking, obesity or alcohol?

BENEFICENCE OF FUTURE PATIENTS VERSUS AUTONOMY AND NON-MALEFICENCE OF PRESENT SUBJECTS

A notice is posted in the Medical School asking for volunteers for a research project. A 'fee' of £50 is being offered. Is the volunteers' autonomy being overridden? Are they being bribed? What are their motives?

It is particularly important when **volunteers** are involved in research that the principle of doing no harm is safeguarded. When patients are involved in the research then there is also the possibility of benefit to them even though there may be the side-effects we referred to above. In most cases, all the ethical principles can be honoured and the benefits maximized by using a careful protocol with independent scrutiny. Autonomy is preserved by the consent process: volunteers and patients have to agree in writing to take part even though there is only a small risk of harm. In many big trials there is an independent data and ethics committee to keep a close eye on the progress and, if any unexpected harm is coming to the subjects, the trial can be stopped or redesigned.

For volunteers to agree to be involved in research shows either a remarkable degree of unselfishness, or a severe shortage of money! It is praiseworthy that they are prepared to accept some risks to themselves for the benefit of other people, but financial incentives add another dimension. However, their autonomy is preserved because of the strict consent process and it is more important then ever that they are told the truth and the

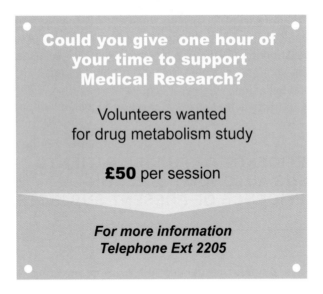

whole truth (as far as it is known) about the treatments and procedures.

There are many other examples that could be used to illustrate the competition between ethical principles and the decisions that have to be made about priority. The challenge in practice is to identify which principles are involved and to analyse the way in which they affect what is being done and this will be the subject of the next chapter.

Summary
- In practice, good ethical principles often compete with each other and one has to be given priority.
- Sometimes the competition can be resolved and all principles honoured by the way the situation is handled.
- Diluting and trying to merge principles is unhelpful.
- Occasionally priority order is changed for a special reason but should be restored as soon as possible.
- Emotional overtones can sometimes cloud clear ethical thinking.

13

FORMING ETHICAL PATHWAYS

It is one thing to be familiar with ethical decisions that have been made in the past and to understand case law, but quite another to be able to analyse and make sense of new ethical problems. These will continue to arise for as long as medicine progresses and human beings have moral codes. However the essential ethical ingredients of the dilemmas are usually the same but in a different guise and in a different context. Pathways for ethical analysis and decision-making for any clinical or research situation will now be addressed.

KEY QUESTION

Which value system undergirds the ethics?

We have stressed in Chapter 4 that different value systems influence the basis of ethical decisions. Therefore, each person should be sure of his or her beliefs and values. Often, different value systems will lead to the same decisions, but sometimes they may result in significant differences (Figure 14.1, page 161).

PRELIMINARY QUESTIONS (FIGURE 13.1)

1. Is the overall aim ethical?

The answer to this question in health care is, of course, usually 'yes'; but the question needs to be asked. For example, research into germ warfare or the development of a new expensive operation when there is already a safe, established alternative, should raise doubts.

2. Are there myths or misunderstandings?

At the beginning of any analysis we must clarify the questions that are being asked and the precise issues involved. For example, if the son of an elderly patient with acute peritonitis says 'You will let her slip away peacefully during the operation won't you doctor?', the surgeon needs to clarify exactly what is meant! Is the doctor being asked to undertake active euthanasia? Is the son unhappy with the decision to operate at all? Or is he worried that the patient may be on a life support machine in intensive care for weeks after the operation? Is the son a beneficiary of the will?!

3. Who and what are involved?

Many ethical problems affect several different groups of people. *In vitro* fertilization (IVF), for example, involves a woman, her long-term partner, possibly a sperm donor and embryos; fertilization and storage techniques and are also involved. There is no ethical problem with a husband fertilizing his wife's ova and the technique of IVF is well established even though the re-implantation cannot be guaranteed to be successful. However, donor semen involves a third person, even though he is initially anonymous, and spare embryos create a significant ethical problem for some people.

Figure 13.1 Algorithm illustrating the preliminary questions to ask

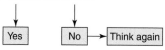

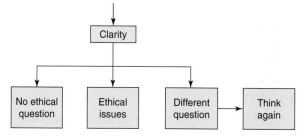

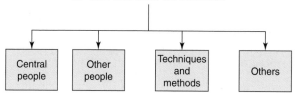

ETHICAL ANALYSIS (FIGURE 13.2)

4. Which ethical principles are involved?

Using the example of IVF, the following principles are involved:

- Autonomy of the couple and the 'right' to have a child.
- The husband's and donor's autonomy.
- Beneficence to the couple and their family.
- Maleficence to spare embryos if they are destroyed.
- Confidentiality of the donor.
- Justice and equity, if NHS resources are used.
- Truth: they need to be fully informed of the chances of success.

5. Are any of these in competition?

At least three pairs of competing principles can be seen:

- Beneficence for the couple and maleficence to spare embryos. The importance of this will depend on one's view of the value of embryos.
- Autonomy of the couple versus justice to other couples and other patients in the Health Service.
- The confidentiality of the donor versus the autonomy of the unborn child.

6. Can they be resolved by changing methods or techniques?

Often they can. In this example, as techniques for fertilization and implantation improve, a single embryo implantation will become the norm, reducing the need for spare embryos. Second, the autonomy versus justice issue is resolved by limiting IVF attempts on the NHS to one or two for each couple (although in some parts of the UK it is still difficult to have any at all).

7. Should one principle take priority?

If the competition cannot be resolved, one principle has to be given priority according to the hierarchies in Chapter 12. For

Figure 13.2 Algorithm illustrating ethical analysis

4. Which ethical principles are involved?

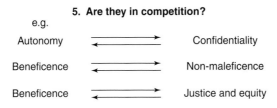

5. Are they in competition?

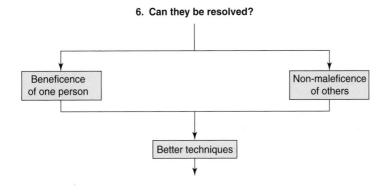

6. Can they be resolved?

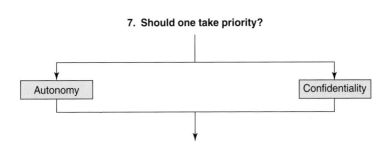

7. Should one take priority?

years, in law, the confidentiality of the donor has taken priority over the autonomy of the child, but no longer (see question 10).

8. What are the likely long-term consequences that have an ethical dimension?

Any research project can produce unexpected side-effects, otherwise it would not be true research. The question is whether the design should be altered or the research stopped. In 2006, six normal volunteers in London developed multi-organ failure during a phase 1 drug trial and spent many days in intensive care.

FURTHER CHECKS (FIGURE 13.3)

9. Is there already professional guidance?

In the case of IVF, the Human Fertilisation and Embryology Authority (HFEA) lays down clear guidelines about the function ethics of the IVF centres in the UK (HFEA, 2006). The General Medical Council (GMC) and other professional groups give written guidance on confidentiality.

10. Is there legal guidance?

Before making an ethical decision we need to check statute law and case law as well as guidance from statutory authorities. In the case of IVF, the HFEA, in the sixth edition of its code of practice, has recently reversed the priority given to the confidentiality of the donor. Children born through IVF now have the right to meet their genetic father when they reach the age of 18.

11. Should the problem be referred to a research or clinical ethics committee?

If there is a research element then it must be referred to the research ethics committee. If there are unusual circumstances or variations from standard procedure it is advisable to get advice

Figure 13.2 (Continued)

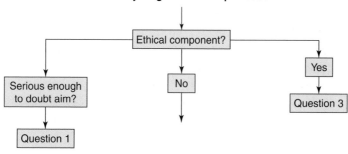

8. Likely long-term consequences?

Figure 13.3 Algorithm illustrating further checks to be made

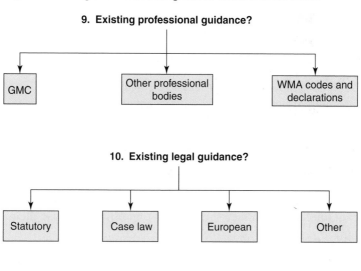

9. Existing professional guidance?

10. Existing legal guidance?

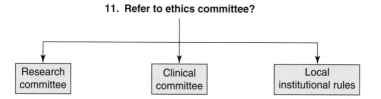

11. Refer to ethics committee?

from a clinical ethics committee or group before proceeding. In addition many hospitals have local policies and procedures.

12. Will the decision start a precedent?

When controlling legislation is already in place then a decision is unlikely to set a precedent, but if the decision is determined by case law, then future cases may be governed by this precedent. The much-derided 'slippery slope' is a reality, especially if laws or policies are not tightly worded. The 1967 Abortion Law is a good example of this (for further discussion, see Chapter 6). Ethical consistency is important.

13. Is the rest of the care team happy with the ethical decisions?

Care is now provided by a multidisciplinary team and it is often difficult for the leader of the team to be aware of all the members' views. For example, a decision on whether to place a 'Do Not Attempt Resuscitation' (DNAR) order may be made by the consultant but the nurse looking after the patient may have different views. If physician-assisted suicide were legalized, one could anticipate sharp disagreements between members of the same team unless an appointment to a post was conditional on agreeing to a policy (which might contravene the human rights of the individual).

Disagreements can sometimes be resolved by debate and discussion. However, if no consensus is reached, the head of the team might have to take the decision and others exercise their right to act according to their consciences.

14. Has anyone discussed it with the patient?

Often, the patient is the last to hear about a decision affecting his or her health! For example, for years DNAR orders were decided by the doctors without any reference to the patients themselves.

In the next chapter we will apply these algorithms to a variety of different examples.

Figure 13.3 (Continued)

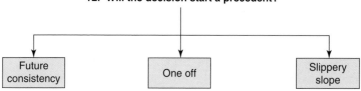

12. Will the decision start a precedent?

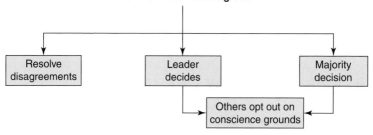

13. Do rest of team agree?

14. Has anyone discussed it with the patient?

14

ETHICAL PATHWAYS
IN PRACTICE

We will now apply the algorithms presented in Chapter 13
to specific examples from different areas of medical practice
and will outline the broad steps in the decision-making
process.

EXAMPLE 1: A NEW OPERATION

*A surgeon plans to perform a laparoscopic ('key-hole') major
liver resection on a man with a tumour. He has done many
open liver resections and many laparoscopic cholecystectomies
before but not this particular procedure. It is the first time it
has been performed in this country although it is established in
a few centres in other European countries.*

Key question
Which value system?

Systems that value medical progress above the individual will
have a different perspective from those that value all people
equally (see Figure 14.1).

Figure 14.1 Diagram illustrating the key question about value systems

Which value system?

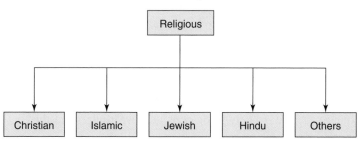

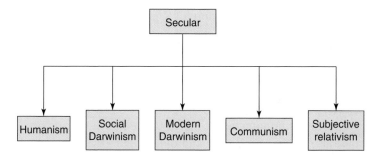

Preliminary questions (see Figure 14.2)

1. Is the overall aim ethical?

Although the declared overall aim is to benefit the patient, it is easy for other aims to creep in, such as prestige, attracting patient referrals, increasing private practice and the excitement of a technical challenge.

2. Are there myths or misunderstandings?

An aura of magic hangs around so-called 'keyhole surgery', with many patients unclear about what is actually involved. The differences from open surgery are a smaller wound and a potentially quicker recovery and discharge from hospital. The time in theatre is likely to be considerably longer, and the operation may be more expensive.

3. Who and what are involved?

The patient, the surgeon and the whole surgical team are involved. The technique involves special instruments and working from a two-dimensional TV monitor with its intrinsic deficiencies.

Ethical analysis (see Figure 14.3)

4. Which ethical principles are involved?

The patient's autonomy and consent to the new operation are important, as are beneficence and non-maleficence – the benefits and risks of such a procedure. Confidentiality only comes into the equation if the surgeon appears on the local TV station that evening to announce the team's achievement! Justice and equity are only involved if this procedure takes much more money or theatre time and therefore stops other people having the operation they need. Truth and integrity present a real challenge: does the surgeon say that this is the first time he has performed this particular procedure or does he concentrate on his experience in other laparoscopic surgery and liver surgery?

Figure 14.2 Algorithm illustrating the preliminary questions to ask

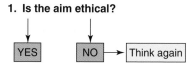

1. Is the aim ethical?

YES   NO → Think again

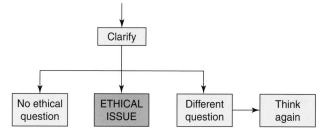

2. Myths or misunderstandings?

Clarify

No ethical question   ETHICAL ISSUE   Different question → Think again

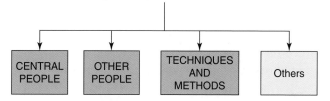

3. Who and what are involved?

CENTRAL PEOPLE   OTHER PEOPLE   TECHNIQUES AND METHODS   Others

Figure 14.3 Algorithm illustrating ethical analysis

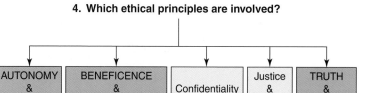

4. Which ethical principles are involved?

AUTONOMY & CONSENT   BENEFICENCE & NON-MALEFICENCE   Confidentiality   Justice & fairness   TRUTH & INTEGRITY

Should he also say it is the first time it has been done in this country?

5. Are any of these in competition?

There may be competition between the following pairs:

- Beneficence v. non-maleficence. There is a possible benefit but a greater risk during the operation of damaging other structures or of complications resulting from a longer anaesthetic.
- Autonomy of this patient v. benefit to future patients. This patient is something of a 'guinea pig' for the possible benefit of future patients.
- Consent v. truth. If the surgeon tells the patient the facts it is possible that the patient will withhold consent.

6. Can they be resolved by changing methods or techniques?

Resolution depends mainly on the careful way the surgeon talks to the patient and gains his confidence. To reduce risk, the surgeon must have studied the operation and trained with an expert abroad. Ideally, he will be assisted by such an expert as a mentor during this procedure. Benefit to future patients largely depends on this patient's altruism and how much he is prepared to be a pioneer.

7. Should one principle take priority?

Patient autonomy takes priority and it must not be subordinated to the surgeon's ambitions. The patient must not be pressurized into agreeing by 'spin'. If telling the patient the truth leads to refusal of consent – so be it.

Figure 14.3 (Continued)

5. Are they in competition?

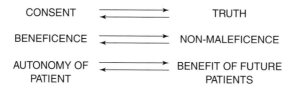

CONSENT   TRUTH

BENEFICENCE   NON-MALEFICENCE

AUTONOMY OF PATIENT   BENEFIT OF FUTURE PATIENTS

6. Can they be resolved?

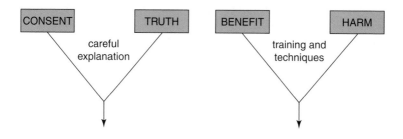

CONSENT   TRUTH   BENEFIT   HARM

careful explanation   training and techniques

7. Should one take priority?

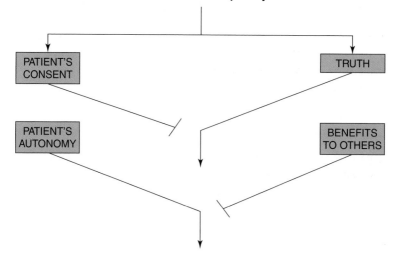

PATIENT'S CONSENT   TRUTH

PATIENT'S AUTONOMY   BENEFITS TO OTHERS

8. What are the likely long-term consequences that have an ethical dimension?

This procedure is unlikely to lead to long-term consequences with an ethical dimension.

Further checks (see Figure 14.4)

9. Is there already professional guidance?

Unlike new drugs, new operations do not have to be licensed in this country. However, since 2002, the National Institute for Health and Clinical Excellence (NICE) has been responsible for the safety and efficacy of new interventional procedures. Many new procedures are only performed under the conditions of a controlled trial so that their true worth can be assessed. General professional guidance emphasizes that a surgeon undertaking any procedure must have adequate assistance.

10. Is there legal guidance?

Drug licensing is by a statutory committee advising the Secretary of State for Health. In the case of an individual operation, if something goes wrong a surgeon can be sued and would be judged under the Bolam and Bolitho tests of what a reasonable body of medical opinion would have done and what a patient could reasonably expect.

11. Should the problem be referred to a research or clinical ethics committee?

As it is not pure research it does not have to be referred to the research ethics committee, but most hospitals either have a clinical ethics committee to which such questions can be referred or have established policy and procedure for the introduction of new techniques.

Figure 14.3 (Continued)

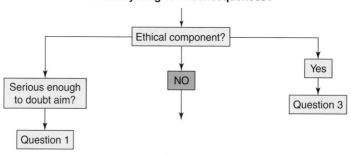

8. **Likely long-term consequences?**

Figure 14.4 Algorithm illustrating further checks to be made

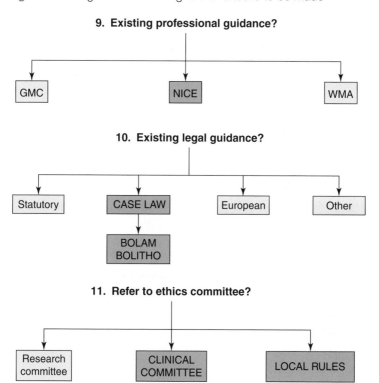

9. **Existing professional guidance?**

10. **Existing legal guidance?**

11. **Refer to ethics committee?**

12. Will the decision start a precedent?

The decision about a case like this could easily lead to a precedent for other new operations. Indeed, when laparoscopic cholecystectomy was first introduced in the UK during the 1980s, there was almost a 'free-for-all' with surgeons trying out the new method after very little training and without any control. The decision in this case must be such that when any future new operation is introduced, the same procedure is followed so that ethical consistency is established.

13. Is the rest of the care team happy with the ethical decisions?

It is important to realize that the surgeon cannot make the decision by himself and that the whole multidisciplinary team should be involved. There have been many examples when surgeons did things that the nursing staff were not entirely happy about, which puts them in a very difficult position. It is important to discuss this beforehand, not once the operation has started!

14. Has anyone discussed it with the patient?

This is essential, of course, but the timing is quite important. If the patient is told all about the possibility of an operation before the procedure is set up this can lead to him being disappointed if it does not go ahead. On the other hand, it must not all be arranged and then just mentioned to him at the last minute with the theatre porters waiting outside the ward with their trolley!

N.B. For the subsequent examples, the same figures apply (see chapter 13, pages 153–157).

Figure 14.4 (Continued)

12. Will the decision start a precedent?

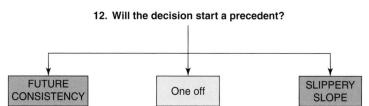

13. Do rest of team agree?

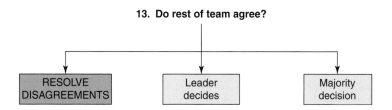

14. Has anyone discussed it with the patient?

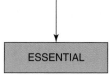

EXAMPLE 2: SAVIOUR SIBLINGS

The parents of a child with thalassaemia want to use pre-implantation genetic diagnosis (PGD) in order to select an embryo for implantation that is an ideal donor for an existing sibling with a very specific serious condition. PGD enables doctors to identify the human leukocyte antigen (HLA) of an embryo produced by in vitro *fertilization (IVF).*

Key question

Which value system?

In this case the value system will have a marked influence on the conclusions because the procedure involves discarding 'unsuitable' embryos (see Figure 14.1, page 161).

Preliminary questions (see Figure 13.1, page 153)

1. Is the overall aim ethical?

There is no doubt that the overall motive is one of compassion and the aim is to help the patient with a serious, non trivial, disease. Most philosophies would agree that helping another human being is good.

2. Are there myths or misunderstandings?

It is easy for a subject like this to become emotive, especially if given extensive media publicity. The child is not being produced **solely** to treat the sibling and then to be discarded or not wanted. Presumably the parents would like a second child, but one free of thalassaemia who could also help his or her sister. Hopefully, the child would be specially valued. In large families there is a good chance that there may already be a sibling with compatible HLA.

3. Who and what are involved?

This complex problem involves parents, existing child, unborn child, embryos, DNA technology, selection and implantation.

Ethical analysis (see Figure 13.2, page 155)

4. Which ethical principles are involved?

In this case the following principles are involved:

- The autonomy of the unborn child, who cannot give consent.
- Beneficence to the existing child.
- Non-maleficence to discarded embryos.
- Safety of selected embryo, as techniques are relatively new.
- Truth relates to a realistic understanding of the risks and chances of success.

5. Are any of these in competition?

Beneficence to the child patient competes with both the destruction of embryos and the autonomy of the sibling yet to be born, who cannot consent to being a donor.

6. Can they be resolved by changing methods or techniques? and 7. Should one principle take priority?

For those who believe that human life starts at fertilization (rather than implantation or later) the issues are unresolvable because they would consider it equivalent to killing many human beings in order to save one. For those, by contrast, who believe that life begins at implantation or birth, the benefit to the value of the existing child outweighs the destruction of embryos. The autonomy of the unborn child is more difficult, and that resolution depends on attitudes and careful explanation as he or she is growing up; however, the child's autonomy cannot be given back after the event.

8. What are the likely long-term consequences that have an ethical dimension?

There are several in this case. The new child might turn out not to be the ideal donor. Would the child therefore not be valued by the parents? In the future the new sibling could be asked to donate other organs, but that also applies to siblings in other families born after natural fertilization. The long-term effects of bone marrow transplantation need to be monitored carefully. The emotional relationship between the siblings could create long-term psychological problems if not handled with care.

Further checks (see Figure 13.3, page 157)

9. Is there already professional guidance?

The ethics of these issues is still under debate within the profession. Control is clearly under the HFEA, but its decisions have already been challenged in court.

10. Is there legal guidance?

There are at least three cases where similar decisions have been made:

- Hashmi 2001. A licence was given by HFEA but then revoked by the High Court on the grounds that PGD must only be used in the interests of the child to be conceived. The High Court decision was overturned in the Court of Appeal in 2003 and the Pro-Life Alliance then went to the House of Lords to review the Court of Appeal's decision. The House of Lords upheld the Court of Appeal's decision but, by this time, Mrs Hashmi was nearly 40 years old.
- Whitakers 2002. The licence was refused by the HFEA. This was refused on the grounds that the unborn child should not be exposed to the hazards of PGD without direct benefit to itself. The parents travelled to Chicago for PGD treatment.
- Fletchers 2004. The HFEA relaxed the rules and licensed PGD in the case of this child.

The first child had thalassaemia and the other two had Diamond Blackfan anaemia – both severe conditions.

11. Should the problem be referred to a research or clinical ethics committee?

This is not relevant because of the role of the HFEA.

12. Will the decision start a precedent?

There is understandable anxiety that a decision to allow this particular form of selection could lead to all sorts of 'designer babies' with special characteristics requested by the parents. It could also lead to PGD for trivial rather than severe diseases. However the HFEA have not given 'carte blanche' but will look at each case on its individual merit and has stressed that PGD should be a last resort.

EXAMPLE 3: CLINICAL TRIALS

In the USA a randomized, placebo-controlled trial was performed to see whether the transplantation of foetal nigral cells into the brain was really effective in the treatment of Parkinson's disease. A placebo group went through the whole procedure but did not have the cells implanted. This involved two operations under general anaesthetic with magnetic resonance imaging (MRI) stereotactic frame, burr holes and cyclosporin to prevent rejection. Apart from the surgeon, all the staff involved and the patients were blinded to (did not know) who was having the cells implanted and who was not. There was heated correspondence in the medical press about the ethics of such an invasive placebo procedure. It was a daring trial!

Key questions
Which value system?

As in the previous example, attitudes to the value of the foetus again will be critical because foetal cells were taken from aborted foetuses and anti-abortion groups were strongly against. However, taking tissue from spontaneous miscarriages would probably be more acceptable if it was technically possible (see Figure 14.1, page 161).

Preliminary questions (see Figure 13.1, page 153)

1. Is the overall aim ethical?

The aim is to treat people with a distressing disease, but also to ensure that patients are not subjected to expensive, invasive treatments if these are not effective. Patients can be psychologically affected if they are given false hopes or spend their own money on useless procedures.

2. Are there myths or misunderstandings?

Patients can easily be misled by apparently miraculous cures. This was the very reason that the trial was undertaken. The 'drama' of an invasive procedure must be balanced against the 'routine' of drug treatment.

3. Who and what are involved?

Two groups of patients with the same condition, half of whom will receive the treatment and half of whom will not. Surgeons, anaesthetists, nurses and other professional staff are all involved. Also involved are aborted foetuses, intricate techniques to locate the exact site in the brain, and powerful drugs with side-effects.

Ethical analysis (see Figure 13.2, page 155)

4. Which ethical principles are involved?

Autonomy and consent are fundamental to such a trial and in any such study there is the balance of beneficence and non-maleficence – benefit and harm. Truth and integrity on behalf of the team are vital if the patient's autonomy is to be preserved, and the surgeons will have to keep the promises they have made to the patients in the future.

5. Are any of these in competition?

If the doctors already knew that the control (placebo) group would suffer from not having the operation, the trial would have been unethical. If they genuinely did not know, that is, they had equipoise, they were **obliged** to do the trial. The integrity of those assessing the outcomes could be under threat if they knew which treatment each patient was given. Power calculations must be done to ensure that enough patients are studied to get a meaningful result, otherwise the trial is unethical because patients have been put at some risk without the possibility of obtaining an answer. Consent could only have been given if the patients agreed that they might or might not receive the active treatment: they had to be informed that they were part of this sort of placebo trial. Finally there is direct competition between the harm to the foetuses and benefit to the patients.

6. Can they be resolved by changing methods or techniques?

Most of the conflicts can be resolved by careful design of the trial. The concern about doing harm (or failing to do good) to the control (placebo) group was overcome, first by continuing the anti-Parkinson's drugs in both groups and second, by promising all participants that if the results of the treatment were positive, the control group would receive the active treatment immediately.

7. Should one principle take priority?

For some, the obligation not to harm the foetuses would take precedence over helping the patients, but for others the reverse argument would hold.

8. What are the likely long-term consequences that have an ethical dimension?

This question is part of the reason for the trial. The side-effects were largely unknown and the follow-up had to be long. If

unexpected serious side-effects were discovered later, then the
ethics of the treatment would be in question.

Further checks (see Figure 13.3, page 157)

9. Is there already professional guidance?

The World Medical Association's Declaration of Helsinki is the
blueprint for the ethics of clinical trials of all types which involve
human subjects (Declaration of Helsinki, 1964). In this trial
patients in both groups are having their disease treated; normal
volunteers are not included as this would have raised further
questions. In the UK, the Medical Research Council (MRC) has
given advice on consent for research procedures. In 2004, the
Central Office for Research Ethics Committees (COREC) published
New Standard Operating Procedures for Research Ethics
Committees and, in the same year, the European Union Directive
on Clinical Trials of Medicinal Products came into force.

10. Is there legal guidance?

The law on valid consent applies in this case. In 2004, UK
Clinical Trials Regulations were established in the form of the
Medicines for Human Use (Clinical Trials) Regulations 2004.

11. Should the problem be referred to a research or clinical ethics committee?

Yes this type of study would have to go to the institutional
research ethics committee. In the event it was approved.

12. Will the decision start a precedent?

Placebo-controlled trials are commonly used in evaluating drugs
and have previously been used in some surgical and other interventional procedures. Use of foetal cells could create a precedent.

13. Is the rest of the care team happy with the ethical decisions?

There are many different groups of professionals involved. For
example the theatre nurses would have to agree to help with

the operation. Those doing the objective assessment would also have to be happy with the protocol even though they were not actually doing the procedure.

14. Has anyone discussed it with the patient?

If they had not, the whole trial would have been unethical! The ethics committee would want to approve the exact wording of the consent form which was used to ensure that the patients were being fully informed.

Result

The interesting and unexpected result of this trial was that the placebo group did better than the treatment group! The latter developed unforeseen complications due to scarring at the site of implantation. Even though this result justified performing the trial, it was still important that each stage was designed to be ethical. Many patients have probably been prevented from having an expensive and ineffective, if not harmful, treatment because these patients agreed to be involved.

EXAMPLE 4: MANAGEMENT OF COMMUNICABLE DISEASES

HIV/AIDS affects millions of people world-wide and was dubbed the 'twentieth-century plague'. The incidence continues to rise throughout the world, leaving hundreds of thousands of orphans and decimating the young population of many developing countries.

Key question

Which value system?

Choice of value system may well influence some ethical decisions in this area, because the spread of infection is related to the morality of lifestyles (see Figure 14.1, page 161).

Preliminary questions (see Figure 13.1, page 153)

1. Is the overall aim ethical?

There is general agreement that to try to prevent, control and even cure such a devastating disease is good and ethical. Other less worthy aims might creep in, such as making substantial profits from manufacturing and distributing drugs or condoms, often in very poor countries. Worthiness of the aim, for those who are not utilitarian, does not necessarily justify all methods of control and treatment.

2. Are there myths or misunderstandings?

There are many misunderstandings concerning the spread and treatment of HIV. One of the most devastating is the belief, in some cultures, that it can be cured by having sex with a young virgin. Another is the obligation for a man to have sex with his dead brother's wife. There has also been a tendency in some countries to deny that the problem exists and for many people there is a naive trust in the efficacy of condoms to prevent spread of the disease.

3. Who and what are involved?

There is a very long list: governments and health authorities, international drug and vaccine companies, patients, partners, spouses, children, prostitutes, pimps, economic problems, teachers, health promoting agencies and, not least, the many devoted doctors and nurses who are caring for the patients and their relatives.

Ethical analysis (see Figure 13.2, page 155)

4. Which ethical principles are involved?

Autonomy, beneficence, confidentiality and justice are the most important ingredients. There is also an issue of the autonomy of the health care team who themselves may be put at risk of infection.

5. Are any of these in competition?

The issue of confidentiality of a patient is a direct challenge to the rights (autonomy) of partners and contacts. As discussed in Chapter 10 it may be right to break confidentiality in special circumstances to prevent harm to an individual. Second, the patient's right only to be HIV-tested with consent and to have sexual partners as and when he or she likes is in direct competition with the health of others, even if they are willing partners. Because patients can only be tested with their express consent, we do not know the real size of the problem.

6. Can they be resolved by changing methods or techniques? and 7. Should one principle take priority?

Is it possible to compel people to alter their behaviour for the benefit of other people's health? A total smoking ban in public places in the UK comes near to this, but it is difficult to see how sexual activity could be regulated in the same way! The difference is that people usually choose to be sexual partners, but they do not choose to be passive smokers. Persuasion can help and providing needles and syringes to drug addicts to reduce needle-sharing is a good example. (For a discussion of compulsory and voluntary screening for HIV, see Beauchamp and Childress, 2001, page 277ff.)

Uganda was the first country to reduce the rise in HIV; they have done this by an intensive educational programme based on A B C – abstain, be faithful and use condoms if necessary. This method still leaves patients with their autonomy intact while asking them to curtail it for the sake of themselves and others. At present, in the UK, confidentiality overrides risks to other people even though patients are persuaded to tell their partners and contacts to get in touch with the STD clinic. Whether confidentiality should have such a priority over the health of others is still a moot point.

8. What are the likely long-term consequences that have an ethical dimension?

Future management will involve more effective drugs and hopefully vaccines. The long-term implication may well be a relaxation of behaviour once the fear of contracting HIV has gone. This may lead to an increase in other sexually transmitted disease or diseases spread via needles, such as hepatitis C, for which there is at present little effective treatment. This has an ethical component as does the issue of distributive justice. There will be a great problem ensuring that patients have access to new treatments in the poorest countries of the world.

Further checks (see Figure 13.3, page 157)

9. Is there already professional guidance?

The GMC has given specific guidance on confidentiality and other issues in their publication *Serious Communicable Diseases* (GMC, 1997). This advises that often the problem can be overcome by careful and open discussion with the patient but, in particular cases the health care team should be told if there is a serious risk to them. In wealthy countries it is possible to use universal precautions to protect the staff but even rubber gloves are in very short supply in developing countries.

10. Is there legal guidance?

The key legal guidance was the decision not to make AIDS a notifiable disease under the Public Health (Control of Diseases) Act of 1984, thereby protecting the patient's confidentiality.

11. Should the problem be referred to a research or clinical ethics committee?

Should a doctor deem it necessary to break confidentiality and tell a patient's partner because of the specific risk to him or her, it is wise to discuss it with senior colleagues. If clinical trials of new drugs are performed, these should go to the ethics committee in the normal way.

12. Will the decision start a precedent?

Variation in response to different infectious diseases has already been mentioned. If somebody is suspected of having severe acute respiratory syndrome (SARS) or bird flu they can immediately be isolated and forbidden to travel. Yet no such restrictions are put on a disease that is already killing millions. When vaccination becomes available can it and should it be made compulsory for certain groups of people?

13. Is the rest of the care team happy with the ethical decisions?

It has been pointed out that there are large numbers of people involved in grappling with this devastating problem from many different ethnic, cultural and religious backgrounds and it would not be at all surprising if disagreements on particular management strategies arose.

14. Has anyone discussed it with the patient?

It is easy, when conducting large studies, to ignore the individual patient.

CONCLUSION

This chapter has demonstrated how to make sense of the ethics of four different examples. Not all the questions are equally relevant to each situation, but they provide a useful aid to focus on the important ethical questions and to ensure that difficult decisions are not ignored or avoided. Difficulties and confusions often arise because the issues are not identified, clarified and made explicit.

15

ETHICS SURVIVAL GUIDE FOR MEDICAL STUDENTS

Student doctors are in the unique position of being a hybrid of a lay person and a professional. You may think of yourself as a lay person but doctors may expect you to be professional. Patients very often assume that you have more knowledge and ability than you actually have and may relate to you more easily than to the qualified doctors. Sometimes you are taking a history or taking blood as part of the care team and at other times you are merely an observer. This odd situation raises a number of ethical concerns about the role you should have in the hospital and what information you should give to patients and relatives. Students who do not know what to do in an uncomfortable situation often adopt a policy of silence. This can happen because they feel unsure about the distinction between acceptable and unacceptable behaviour, or, when learning practical procedures, are unsure how much they are allowed to do. It is important to recognize these concerns and deal with them as they arise. If you can decide where you stand on certain issues you are less likely to grow cynical through feeling that you cannot speak out.

Patients are often your teachers. There is no way in which medicine can be learnt without having frequent contact with them. It is also important to remember that doctors and nurses are also there to help you learn. Sometimes your ignorance is exposed in front of a patient which can be embarrassing, and here we discuss some of the situations that you may find awkward or difficult.

PATIENTS' HISTORIES AND DIAGNOSES

It is one of the extraordinary privileges of being in medicine that patients trust us enough to tell us the most intimate details of their lives, and confidentiality is fundamental to the process (see Chapter 9). Sometimes, however, patients may say to a student 'If I tell you this you won't tell the doctors will you'?

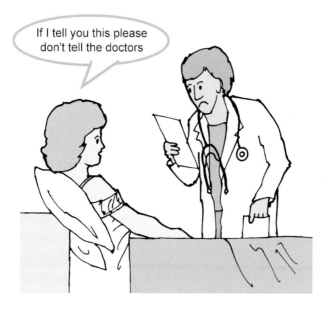

It is even more difficult if they tell you the details first and then ask you not to pass them on. You have to tell the patient that you cannot make that promise if the information has an important bearing on his or her health and treatment. If it is a non-relevant piece of information the patient wants to share with you that is different. Patients often tend to feel less intimidated when asking students to explain aspects of their diagnosis and care to them.

Alternatively a patient might suddenly ask you about his or her diagnosis by saying 'I didn't want to bother the doctors as they are so busy'. If you do not know the diagnosis or the results of a recent biopsy, you can honestly say that you do not know. If you **do** know, this is more difficult as it is not your role to discuss diagnosis and prognosis and you probably do not have **all** the facts. You can safely say that you do not know all the facts and that you will ask the doctor to come and discuss things with the patient.

> Never tell a lie or invent something to reassure a patient.

SITTING IN ON A CONSULTATION

Students regularly sit in on consultations in hospital or general practice and can feel awkward or redundant in this situation. Being involved with the patient by taking a history or helping in some way is far easier than just being an observer. The normal ethical practice is for the doctor to ask patients if they mind a student being present, and usually there is no problem. If a patient declines then you are in the awkward position of having to leave. However this does not mean that students should not be present at difficult or distressing consultations: it is very important to learn from them, especially if there is an opportunity to discuss them afterwards.

The majority of patients have no problem with one or two students being present but they do not like being gazed at by a crowd! Most clinics will have a notice in the waiting room saying there are students in the clinic and asking patients to mention it beforehand if they do not wish them to be present. This avoids an awkward situation.

In general practice, especially if you live in the same city, make sure that patients know your name before the consultation so that there is not an embarrassing encounter between you and a close friend's mother! In any consultation it can be difficult for a student to know whether to ask questions in front of a patient or not. If in doubt, it is wiser to wait until afterwards.

CHAPERONES

Examining a patient of the opposite sex always has the potential for problems and the tradition of chaperones is to protect the student and doctor as much as the patient. All groups of students are now mixed sex so it is easy for students to help each other by examining in pairs. If no chaperone is available, you should return on another occasion.

PRACTICAL PROCEDURES

However much you have practised on mannequins, procedures such as venepuncture have to be learnt on patients eventually. It is important to explain to patients what you are doing and why, and obtain verbal and implied consent. It is equally important that you do not give the patient unnecessary discomfort. If you fail repeatedly, as you may, you should not persist but, instead, ask a house officer or SHO to take over. Other procedures (e.g. catheterization) you may do under direct guidance from a doctor with the patient being aware and having consented to a 'teaching procedure'.

A group of students in a leading teaching hospital were told by the consultant when they started a surgical attachment to ask for help if they failed to obtain blood, rather than persist with venepuncture. Before long, one student approached the consultant saying that he had a problem with obtaining blood from an elderly patient. He was congratulated on taking the advice seriously but, as they entered the room the cause was obvious – the patient was dead!

Common sense can help in many situations; it was Mark Twain who quipped that, sadly, there was not enough of it around to be common! Assisting a surgeon in the operating theatre is not just being involved in patient care, but should also be a good learning experience. However, clearly it is important that a student does what is asked rather than acting independently.

LEARNING INTIMATE EXAMINATIONS

In the 'bad old days' students used to learn how to do rectal and vaginal examinations on unconscious patients in the operating theatre without their consent. This was not ethical because it broke the principle of autonomy; consent for the operation did not include consent for other people to do 'unnecessary' examinations. But students must learn these techniques or serious errors of diagnosis will be made in the future. Nowadays there are mannequins on which techniques can initially be learnt and skills tested during examinations, but speaking to a mannequin as if it is a living person is a strange experience! After the initial skills are mastered, conscious patients can be asked to give their consent for one or two students to perform an examination under instruction.

RESEARCH PROJECTS

You may be asked to be involved in helping to run clinical research projects, in which case you must be certain that they are ethical and comply with the Helsinki Declaration and other guidelines.

You might also be approached by a more senior member of your team to be involved as a subject in his or her research. This is in fact unethical because you are in a position where you are being coerced by a person to whom you are in some sense answerable and therefore your co-operation is not entirely of your own free will. Should you be put 'on the spot', you should not agree immediately, but give yourself time to discuss it with others. The correct procedure is for an advert to be placed inviting people to participate and giving a contact number. However, the issue of payment is important because a large payment could act as a bribe and, as most students are hard up, this could be considered to be inappropriate pressure. Financial rewards should be for the inconvenience, the time taken and be of an appropriate amount (see p. 149).

RESPECT FOR THE DEAD

In many medical schools, in the past, the first patient a student saw was a dead one in the dissecting room. Although nowadays, most medical schools ensure contact with live patients early in the course, students will still work with dead bodies at many stages in their studies. It is easy to become very familiar and even flippant, with dead body parts, but it is important for students to learn to respect the dead.

Respect for dead bodies arises from respect for the people they represent and the fact that they have donated their bodies for you to learn from. Some cultures have problems with dissecting bodies at all, while others encourage students to find out as much as possible about the people and their relatives.

A death on the ward may be stressful for students as it may be a new experience and one which challenges their own attitudes to death and immortality. It is important for students to learn how to handle recent deaths by showing respect for the dead and sensitivity towards the relatives.

SHOULD A STUDENT SPEAK OUT?

Mentors and role models are important for learning and one of the advantages of clinical attachments is that students can observe their seniors closely. For learning ethics, observing and copying are not enough and issues need to be discussed openly. However, at times students may observe or be asked to take part in actions which they think are unethical. What do you do? You have a perfect right to refuse to take part – giving your reasons: but should you go to the extent of 'whistle-blowing' on more senior staff?

Your first response might be to ask for an explanation, as you may well not know the background and details and it may indeed be ethical after all. However, if you are still unhappy, you should go to a senior student or your academic or social tutor for further advice.

PASSING THE EXAMINATION

Questions of ethics are often included in examinations either in the context of clinical cases or in written examinations, or independently through extended matching questions or short answers. They may also be the subject of more in-depth dissertations involving literature searches, or form a station in an OSCE exam (e.g. obtaining consent). It is important to realize that, when debating difficult questions such as abortion, euthanasia, cloning or research projects, your aim is not to reach the same conclusions as the examiner, even if his or her views are well known, but to argue your own case cogently and logically. This involves knowing facts and being able to analyse data as well as expressing opinions. The key facts you should know are listed in Box 15.1 and the analytical skills you will need are listed in Box 15.2.

Box 15.1   Facts you should know

- The nature of medical ethics (Chapter 1)
- Ethical theories (Chapter 3)
- Value systems (your own and others) (Chapter 4)
- Ethical principles (Chapters 7–11)
- Existing guidelines – GMC good practice, BMA, WMA codes and declarations (Chapters 1 and 5)
- Key legislation (Chapter 6 and others) and key legal cases that have governed practice
- Implications of breach of duties.

Box 15.2   Analytical skills you will need

In an examination, you will need to be:

- Able to discuss the relationship between personal ethics and codified and professional ethics and law
- Aware of when there is an ethical component in a clinical situation or research proposal
- Able to identify the ethical principles involved
- Aware of conflict and competition between these principles
- Able to argue the relative importance of each
- Able to relate ethical ideals to non-ideal situations, such as distribution of scarce resources.
- Able to search the ethics literature and find guidance

Communication skills are very important for putting patients at their ease, as well as convincing examiners of your arguments.

CONCLUSION

A medical student's lot is not always an easy one but many problems can be prevented by introducing yourself, even though you are wearing a badge, and clarifying your role in the care team. Examples are 'I am a fourth-year medical student and Dr Jones the consultant has suggested I ask you some questions about your illness before he sees you – is that alright?' or 'I am a second-year medical student and have come to take some blood to test that the various chemicals are at the right level after your recent operation – do you mind?' If the dreaded question comes 'Is this the first time you have done it?' you have to reply honestly, with an answer such as 'Yes, but I have been taught how to do it and will ask for help if there is a problem. I promise I won't turn you into a pin cushion!'

Common sense, sensitivity and putting yourself in the patient's place can anticipate and resolve many difficult situations. If you should have the misfortune to be hospitalized yourself during your time as a student you will learn more about patient care and confidentiality in five days than you would otherwise learn in five years!

WHAT MAKES AN ETHICAL DOCTOR?

The French writer Voltaire (1694–1778) described doctors as 'people who give medicines about which they know little, for illness about which they know less, to people about whom they know nothing'. Voltaire was not impressed by doctors! Two and a half centuries later the *British Medical Journal* invited contributions in answer to the question 'What makes a good doctor?' and received 102 answers from 24 countries listing 70 qualities (Box 16.1) (Tonks, 2002).

Box 16.1 Some qualities of a good doctor		
Well known	**Less expected**	**More searching**
Compassion	Courage	A good spouse
Understanding	Creativity	A good colleague
Empathy	A sense of justice	A good customer at the supermarket
Honesty	Respect	A good driver on the road
Competence	Optimism	
Commitment	Grace	
Humanity		

The patient who told her doctor 'I don't care how much you know, until I know how much you care' is making the same point. But being courteous and sympathetic does not in itself make a doctor ethical. By all accounts Harold Shipman was very kind to his patients and they greatly appreciated his care; but then he killed them. Patients want their surgeons to be friendly and sympathetic but not at the expense of a high level of surgical knowledge and skill: a surgeon shows concern and sympathy to patients principally by doing a first-class operation.

There are about 130 000 doctors in the UK and it is not surprising that in a professional group of this size there should be some who do commit crimes, misuse drugs, are corrupted by money or become mentally ill. Despite the media obsession with doctors' mistakes the great majority of doctors are good and valued by their patients. Patients want to trust their doctors, but they are not content any longer with a blind faith: they want to be empowered and want time to discuss their illnesses without being stampeded into a decision.

Box 16.2 lists the qualities in a doctor that American patients rate most highly, which reflects the greater 'patient power' in that health care system. The last is particularly interesting: most doctors protect themselves behind their professional standing and trappings, and find it difficult to admit ignorance, mistakes or inability to help. Doctors are not all paragons of virtue: they are human beings and human beings make mistakes. Hopefully these are usually minor errors of judgement and do not lead to severe harm to patients.

Box 16.2   American patients' view of doctors (Editorial, 2002)

- Honesty
- Openness
- Responsiveness
- Having one's best interest at heart
- Willingness to be vulnerable without fear of being harmed.

HANDLING MISTAKES

Perhaps the most important attribute of ethical doctors is that they can admit their mistakes and learn from them. The climate created by regular audits should make this easier. *Forgive and Remember* (Bosk, 1979) is the title of a book that gives many examples of how facing errors honestly can improve patient care. After an error, your colleagues, the medical authorities and the patient or relatives may forgive you but can you forgive yourself? It is an advantage to have a world-view that includes forgiveness.

PERSONAL STANDARDS

In Chapter 3 we discussed virtue ethics, which concentrate on the good character of doctors rather than their duties or the consequences of their actions. Doctors who are truthful and honest in normal life and social activity will be the same in their professional work. It is very difficult to put on an ethical veneer every time we put on our white coats! Keeping the five principles of ethical behaviour as a constant reminder is a useful and important check.

- Respect for **autonomy** means that we will let the patient ask questions and be a partner in the decision about his or her treatment.
- The doctor who practises **beneficence** will always ask what is in the patient's best interest and what will bring benefit rather than harm.
- **Confidentiality** will be the hallmark of the doctor–patient relationship, building up trust and respect.
- The doctor who values **truth and integrity** will always answer the patients' questions honestly even if this means admitting ignorance or mistakes.
- The doctor who values **justice** will always attempt to use medical resources equitably and fairly, despite the difficulties.

In all this there are always the challenging questions: What would I want if I were in the patient's shoes? and What must it be like to receive the treatment I am suggesting?

COMPETENCE

Patients want their doctors to be competent in all areas of practice, not just medical knowledge. But where do we set the boundaries? After all, statistically, half of all doctors are of

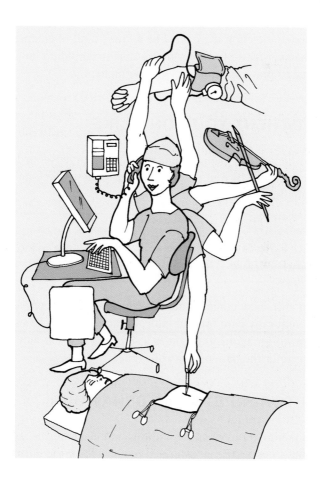

below average competence! Obviously everyone should strive
for excellence but, by definition, excellence is exceptional – it
stands out from the norm. Many formal assessments of clinical
competency may be classified into five levels:

● Excellent
● Good
● Acceptable
● Unacceptable
● Seriously unacceptable.

In the UK the General Medical Council (GMC) would be involved
if the last two are encountered and would take various actions.
For public protection there must be a lower limit of competence
(for whatever reason) below which a doctor should no longer
continue to practise, temporarily or permanently.

THE PATIENT YOU DON'T LIKE

Most clinicians like people: that is why they practise medicine.
But all doctors will find they have a few patients they do not
naturally find easy to accept.

> 'Beware the patient you like very much as well as the one you
> can't stand': there is the danger is that you will make wrong
> decisions for both.

We can still show compassion and concern for someone we
do not naturally care for and ethical practice requires this.
However, if antagonism becomes a serious barrier, it may be
wiser to refer the patient to a colleague.

MONITORING ETHICAL BEHAVIOUR

The British love rules and regulations and every major depart-
ure from good practice produces a report with many new

rules! The problems is that these burden the great majority of doctors who are practising safely and ethically, and probably have little affect on the few who are not. It seems far more important to think positively and do all we can to enhance the good work that is already going on than just concentrate on negative aspects. Another way of helping is to set targets when colleagues appraise each other. However, it is very difficult to assess ethical issues by standard methods. Research protocols can be screened by an ethical committee but whether a doctor gives the right amount of autonomy in a consultation is a much more subtle matter. The problem with medicine, as well as its exciting challenge, is that a doctor cannot just practise by established protocols because new situations will always emerge that demand analysis and the ability to draw on past knowledge and experience in different combinations. Although the disease may be similar, each patient is different and needs to be approached in a way that fits his or her personality.

Maintaining ethical practice needs continued honest self-appraisal as well as checks against external standards and discussion with colleagues.

> *Good doctors are humble doctors, willing to listen to their patients and gather together the full array of resources – medical, human, social and spiritual – that will contribute to their patients' healing.*
>
> (Wolpe, 2002)

MOTIVES MATTER

None of our motives are entirely altruistic, and we may smile at the romantic idealism of the story books; but, in the long term, motives do direct behaviour.

> *'Man has almost limitless ability to convince himself that what he wants to do is morally justifiable'.*
>
> (Smithalls and Beard, 1973)

Here is a list of possible motives in medicine:

- Patient care: an amalgam of professional knowledge gained from tradition, training and experience
- Beliefs: religious and secular
- Curiosity and the quest for knowledge
- Career advancement
- Financial incentives
- The spirit of competition: success, pride and fame
- Pressure from patients and relatives and the fear of litigation.

In Chapter 4 we posed the question: 'Why do we bother to treat sick people at all?' The answer goes to the root of our motives and, therefore, ultimately our ethics. We will end this book with an interesting observation by Roy Hattersley, a self proclaimed atheist writing in the *Guardian* in the aftermath of hurricane Katrina in New Orleans:

> *The Salvation Army has been given a special status as provider-in-chief of American disaster relief. But its work is being augmented by all sorts of other groups. Almost all of them have a religious origin or character. Notable by their absence are teams from rationalist societies, free thinkers' clubs and atheists' associations – the sort of people who not only scoff at religion's intellectual absurdity but also regard it as a positive force for evil. ... The correlation is so clear that it is impossible to doubt that faith and charity go hand in hand.*
>
> (Hattersley, 2005)

FURTHER READING
AND REFERENCES

GENERAL

Books

Beauchamp TL and Childress JF (2001) *Principles of biomedical ethics*, 5th edn. New York: Oxford University Press.

Boyd KM, Higgs R and Pinching A (1997) *New directory of medical ethics*. London: BMJ Books.

Duncan AS, Dunstan GR and Welbourn RB (Eds) (1981) *Dictionary of medical ethics*. London: Darton Longman and Todd.

Gillon R (1985) *Philosophical medical ethics*. Chichester/New York: John Wiley and Son.

Medical Ethics Today (2004) *The BMA handbook of ethics and law*, 2nd edn. London: BMJ Books.

Pojman LP (2006) *Ethics – discovering right and wrong*, 5th edn. Belmont: Thomson Wadsworth.

Journals

Bioethics

Bulletin of Medical Ethics (contains articles, news reviews and comments on all that is happening in the world of medical ethics. www.bullmedeth.info/)

Cambridge Quarterly of Healthcare Ethics

Journal of Clinical Ethics

Journal of Medical Ethics

Journal of Medicine and Philosophy

Kennedy Institute of Ethics Journal

Other regular publications

Christian Medical Fellowship *ethics files*. www.cmf.org.uk/ethics/

Hastings Center *reports*. www.thehastingscenter.org

REFERENCES AND FURTHER READING BY CHAPTER

Sources of further reading are indicated with **.

Preface

Smith J (2005) Ethics education for medical students. *Bull Med Ethics* **208**: 3–4.

Sokol, DK (2005) Meeting the ethical needs of doctors. *BMJ* **330**: 741–742.

Chapter 1

Consensus Statement (1998) Teaching medical ethics and law within medical education: a model for the UK care curriculum. *J Med Ethics* **24**: 188–192.

Dunstan GR (1974) *The artifice of ethics*. London: SCM Press.

**GMC (General Medical Council) (2001) The duties of a doctor registered with the General Medical Council. In *Good medical* *practice*, 3rd edn. London: General Medical Council. www.gmc-uk.org/guidance/

Grenz SJ and Smith JT (2003) *Pocket dictionary of ethics.* Downess Grove, IL: Inter-Varsity Press.

Royal Liverpool Children's Inquiry (2001) *The Report of The Royal Liverpool Children's Inquiry.* www.rlcinquiry.org.uk

The Shipman Inquiry 2005. www.the-shipman-inquiry.org.uk

Chapter 2

Culliford L (2002) Spirituality and clinical care. *BMJ* **325**, 1434–1435.

**Euthanasia debate – for opposing views see: Dignity in Dying. www.Dignityindying.org.uk and Care not Killing. www.carenotkilling.or.uk

GMC (General Medical Council) (2001) The duties of a doctor registered with the General Medical Council. In *Good medical practice*, 3rd edn. London: General Medical Council.www. gmc-uk.org/guidance/

GMC (2002) *Withholding and withdrawing life-prolonging treatments: good practice in decision-making.* London: General Medical Council. www.gmc-uk.org/guidance/

McLean A (1993) *The elimination of morality. Reflections on utilitarianism and bioethics.* London and New York: Routledge.

**National Institute of Health and Clinical Excellence. www.nice.org.uk

Standing Medical Advisory Committee (1996) *The path of least resistance.* London: HMSO.

The Royal College of Psychiatrists (2005) *Spirituality and mental health.* www.rcpsych.ac.uk/info/spirituality.asp

Chapter 3

Anscombe E (1958) Modern moral philosophy. *Philosophy* 33.

Bentham J (1789/1961) *An introduction to the principles of morals and legislation.* Garden City, NY: Doubleday.

Fletcher J (1966) *Situation ethics.* London: SCM Press.

MacIntyre A (1981) *After virtue.* Notre Dame: University of Notre Dame Press.

Mill JS (1861/1998) *Utilitarianism.* New York: Oxford University Press.

Sartre JP (1947) *Existentialism and humanism* (tr. Malnet P 1973). London: Eyre Methuen.

Taylor R (1985) *Ethics faith and reason.* New York: Prentice Hall.

Chapter 4

**Aglouni KM (2003) Values, qualifications, ethics and legal standards in Arabic (Islamic) medicine. *Saudi Med J* 24: 820–826.

**American Humanist Association. www.americanhumanist.org

**Breuilly E, O'Brien J, Palmer M (1997) *Religions of the world.* Jordan: Hodder.

**British Humanist Association. www.humanism.org.uk

British Medical Association (BMA) (1995) *Core values survey report.* London: British Medical Association.

**Crawford SC (2003) *Hindu bioethics for the twenty-first century.* Albany, NY: State University of New York Press.

Dawkins R (1976) *The selfish gene.* Oxford: Oxford University Press.

**Geisler NL (1990) *Christian ethics. Options and issues.* Leicester: Apollos.

Gharem I (1981) Islamic medical jurisprudence. *Med Sci Law* **21: 275–287.

Gray J (2002) *Straw dogs*. London: Granta.

Harris J (1985) *The value of life: an introduction to medical ethics*. London: Routledge and Kegan Paul.

Hindu ethics (1996) *Indian Journal of Medical Ethics* **4(4).

Huxley J (Ed.) (1961) *The humanist frame*. London: George, Allen and Unwin.

**Macquarrie J and Childress JF (1990) *New directory of Christian ethics*. Norwich: SCM Canterbury Press.

**Rosner F (1997) *Modern medicine and Jewish ethics*, 2nd edn. New York: Yeshiva University Press.

Sangharakshita BS (1999) *Vision and transformation: an introduction to the Buddha's noble eightfold path*. Birmingham: Windhorse Publications.

Singer P (1993) *Practical ethics*, 2nd edn. Cambridge: Cambridge University Press.

Singer P (1995) *Rethinking life and death*. Oxford: Oxford University Press.

**Wyatt J (1998) *Matters of life and death*. Leicester: Inter-Varsity Press.

Chapter 5

Editorial (1997) Oaths, codes, declarations and conventions. *Bull Med Ethics* **126: 3–4.

Bristol Royal Infirmary Inquiry (2001) *Learning from Bristol: the report of the public inquiry into children's heart surgery at the Bristol Royal Infirmary 1984–1995*. Command Paper: CM 5207. www.bristol-inquiry.org.uk

**GMC (General Medical Council). www.gmc-uk.org

GMC (General Medical Council) (2001) *Good medical practice,* 3rd edn. London: General Medical Council. www.gmc-uk. org/guidance/

GMC (2002a) *Withholding and withdrawing life-prolonging treatments: good practice in decision-making.* London: General Medical Council. www.gmc-uk.org/guidance/

GMC (2002b) *Research: the role and responsibilities of doctors.* London: General Medical Council. www.gmc-uk.org/guidance/

GMC (2004) *Confidentiality: protecting and providing information.* London: General Medical Council. www.gmc-uk.org/guidance/

Gillon R (1985) Medical oaths, declarations and codes. *BMJ (Clin Res Ed)* **290: 1194–1195.

Savulescu J (2006) Conscientious objection in medicine. *BMJ* **332**: 294–297.

**World Medical Association. www.wma.net

Chapter 6

**British and Irish Legal Information Institute (free). www.bailu.org

**British Medical Association. www.bma.org.uk

**Department for Constitutional Affairs. www.dca.gov.uk (for information about UK legislation)

**Foster C (2005) *Elements of medical law.* Chichester: Barry Rose Law Publishers.

**Incorporated Council of Law Reporting. www.lawreports.co. uk (for law reports)

**Lord Woolf (1999) Civil procedure rules. Department of Constitutional Affairs. www.dca.gov.uk/civil/procrules_fin

**Office of Public Sector Information. www.opsi.gov.uk (for information about UK legislation)

Pattinson SD (2006) *Medical Law and Ethics.* London: Sweet and Maxwell.

**Plome A (2005) *The law and ethics of medical research, international bioethics and human rights.* London: Cavendish Publishing.

Walton, Lord (1994) *Hansard*, 9 May, 1345.
**Westlaw UK. www.westlaw.co.uk

Chapter 7

**Callahan DL (1992) When self-determination runs amok. *Hastings Center Report* (March/April).

Churchill LR (1987) *Rationing health care in America: perception and principles of justice.* Indiana: University of Notre Dame Press.

GMC (General Medical Council) (2001) Consent. In *Good medical practice*, 3rd edn. London General Medical Council. www.gmc-uk.org/guidance/

**Doyal L and Tobias JS (Eds) (2001) *Informed consent in medical research.* London: BMJ Books.

Gray J (2002) *Straw dogs.* London: Granta.

Johnson AG (2001) Informed consent and surgical research. In Doyal L and Tobias JS (Eds) *Informed consent in medical research.* London: BMJ Books, p. 194.

Medical Research Council (2005) *Position statement on research regulation and ethics.* London: Medical Research Council. www.mrc.ac.uk/index/publications

Royal Liverpool Children's Inquiry (2001) *The Report of The Royal Liverpool Children's Inquiry.* www.rlcinquiry.org.uk

Wyatt J (1998) *Matters of life and death.* Leicester: Inter-Varsity Press.

Chapter 8

Bostrom N (2005) The fable of the dragon-tyrant. *J Med Ethics* **31**: 275–277.

Cornell E (2005) What was God thinking? Science can't tell. *Time Magazine*, November 14th.

GMC (General Medical Council) (1998) *Seeking patients' consent: the ethical considerations.* London: General Medical Council. www.gmc-uk.org/guidance/ library/consent.asp

Lewis CS (1940/2002) *The problem of pain.* London: Harper Collins.

**World Health Organization. www.who.int

**World Transhumanist Association. www.transhumanism.org

Chapter 9

Declaration of Geneva (1948/1994) Adopted by the General Assembly of the World Medical Association at Geneva, Switzerland, September 1948.

DH (Department of Health) (2004) *Guidelines on confidentiality for children under 16.* www.dh.gov.uk/PolicyandGuidance

**National Confidential Enquiry into Patient Outcome and Death. www.ncepod.org.uk/

**Office of Public Sector Information. www.opsi.gov.uk (for information about UK legislation e.g. Data Protection Act)

Schmitz D and Wiesing U (2006) Just a family medical history. *BMJ* **332**, 297–298.

Chapter 10

Doyal L and Doyal L (1999) The British national health service: a tarnished moral vision? *Health Care Analysis* **7**: 363–376.

Editorial (1997) Health inequality: the UK's biggest issue. *Lancet* **349**: 1185.

Harris J (1995) Double jeopardy and the veil of ignorance – a reply. *J Med Ethics* **21**: 151–157.

**Kant I (1959) *Foundations of metaphysics and morals.* Trans Lewis White Beck. Indianapolis: Bobbs-Merrill Co.

Kelvin R (2005) A middle way for rationing healthcare resources. *BMJ* **330: 1340–1341.

Koot HM (2001) The study of quality of life: concepts and methods. In Koot HM and Wallender JL (Eds) *Quality of life in child and adolescent illness.* New York: Taylor and Frances, pp. 3–21.

Newdick C (2005) Who should we treat? rights, rationing and resources in the NHS. Oxford: Oxford University Press.

Oregon Health Services Commission (2006) *Prioritized list of health services.* www.oregon.gov/DHS/ healthplan/ priorlist/main.shtml

Phillips C and Thompson G (2001) What is a QALY? www. evidence-based-medicine.co.uk

Chapter 11

Edelstein L (1943) *The Hippocratic Oath: Text, translation and interpretation.* Baltimore: Johns Hopkins Press.

GMC (General Medical Council) (2001) The duties of a doctor registered with the General Medical Council. In *Good medical practice*, 3rd edn. London: General Medical Council. www.gmc-uk.org/guidance/

Gray J (2002) *Straw dogs.* London: Granta.

Guinness O (2000) *Time for truth.* Leicester: Inter-Varsity Press.

Huxley HA (1907) *Aphorisms and reflections from the works of TH Huxley.* London: Macmillan.

Chapter 13

**Human Fertilisation and Embryology Authority.www.hfea. gov.uk

Chapter 14

Beauchamp TL and Childress JF (2001) *Principles of biomedical ethics*, 5th edn. New York: Oxford University Press.

**Central Office for Research Ethics Committees. www.corec.org.uk

Declaration of Helsinki (1964) Adopted by the General Assembly of the World Medical Association at Helsinki, Finland, 1964.

GMC (General Medical Council) (1997) *Serious communicable diseases*. London: General Medical Council. www. gmc-uk.org/guidance/

GMC (2002) *Research: the role and responsibilities of doctors*. London: General Medical Council. www.gmc-uk.org/guidance/

**National Institute of Health and Clinical Excellence. www.nice.org.uk

Chapter 16

Editorial (2002) Patients' views of the good doctor (Editorial). *BMJ* **325**: 668–669.

Bosk CL (1979) *Forgive and remember – managing medical failure*. Chicago and London: Chicago University Press.

Hattersley R (2005) Faith does breed charity. *Guardian* 12 September, p. 31.

Smithalls RW and Beard RW (1973) New horizons in medical ethics. *BMJ* **2**: 464.

Tonks A (2002) Summary of responses. *BMJ* **323**: 715.

West M (2002) What's a good doctor, and how can you make one? *BMJ* **325: 669–670.

Wolpe PR (2002)We are trying to make doctors too good. *BMJ* **325**:712.

INDEX